Thin People
Don't Clean
Their Plates

Thin People Don't Clean Their Plates

Simple Lifestyle Choices for Permanent Weight Loss

Based on the *THIN CHOICES*™ Weight Loss Program

Jill Fleming, MS, RD

Inspiration Presentations Press
LaCrosse, Wisconsin

Although the author and publisher have made every effort to ensure the accuracy and completeness of information contained in this book, we assume no responsibility for errors, inaccuracies, omissions, or any inconsistency herein. Any slights of people, places, or organizations are unintentional.

First printing 2005

ISBN 0-9754888-4-8
LCCN 2004106465

ATTENTION CORPORATIONS, UNIVERSITIES, COLLEGES, AND PRO-FESSIONAL ORGANIZATIONS: Quantity discounts are available on bulk purchases of this book for educational, gift purposes, or as premiums for increasing magazine subscriptions or renewals. Special books or book excerpts can also be created to fit specific needs. For information, please contact Inspiration Presentations Press, P.O. Box 3372, LaCrosse, WI 54602-3372; 866-482-1159; fax 608-782-2074; www.ThinChoices.com; email Jill@thinchoices.com.

DEDICATION

This book is dedicated to all of the overweight people in this world who need my help learning how to eat, becoming active, and living like a thin person. I have met many of you over the course of my studies and while teaching and traveling. I hope to reach the rest of you through this book, for you have been living as an overweight person for far too long. Today you can begin living your life as the thin person you know you are meant to be.

I would also like to thank my husband Colin, and children Nikolai, Brigette, and Peter, for sharing their wife and mother during the many hours of research and writing that were involved in completing this book.

AUTHOR'S NOTE

As with all weight-loss programs, you should obtain your physician's permission and seek his or her supervision before and while you are following the advice provided in *Thin People Don't Clean Their Plates*. This is particularly important if you have a medical condition, such as diabetes, high blood pressure, or heart disease. A registered dietitian's counsel is advised as well. The author and publisher disclaim any liability arising directly or indirectly from the use of the *THIN CHOICES*™ program.

All of the thin people who have been quoted in this book have given their permission to share information about their eating, exercise, and lifestyle habits.

TABLE OF CONTENTS

FOREWORD

If you are tired of feeling out of control with your eating roller coaster and are ready to start feeling comfortable with your self-image again, you have chosen the right book. If I could name one person who I thought had *the most* sensible, easy approach to weight management and food it would automatically be Jill Fleming.

When you read this book, you will find yourself constantly thinking (maybe even saying aloud), "This makes sense, I can do this." And you will be excited. You will feel *good* about yourself and the choices you make every day.

I have followed Jill's formula for a balanced food life for more than two years. It is *not* a diet. It is about changing how you look at and perceive yourself and food. Although I only needed to lose 10 pounds, I now realize that I just didn't feel healthy.

The *THIN CHOICES* concepts involve changes that are easy to incorporate into your life. You can eat *anything* that you like. There are only a few simple concepts that you need to remember.

Jill clearly explains what no one else has—*why* I should do the things she asks me to do. I now understand a lot more about how my body functions and I have a deeper respect for it.

This program will work for anyone, regardless of your current weight, age, or gender. Jill's philosophy works. Food will no longer be the enemy. Her strategies are easy to recall when you are faced with making everyday choices.

Jill helps you look at how and why you eat and makes common sense of it all. She gives you all the tools you need to become a *better* you. *Understanding* is the key to achieving your goals and keeping them. Jill will give you that knowledge. It's that simple. Stop feeling out of control and lose those negative self-image thoughts. Jill helped me *look* at how, what, and why I ate in a new light. Never before had I considered her approach.

Now I eat when I am hungry, stop when I feel satisfied, move my body around a few times each week. I am also able to take a compliment about my figure with a sincere, "Thank you." These are a few of the simple steps Jill gives you to help you start becoming a slimmer, healthier, happier you.

Jill is so passionate about her work. She can motivate even a self-proclaimed couch potato like me. Read on to start an exciting, simple transformation that will make you feel good about what and how you eat.

Go on; start taking care of one of the most important people in your life—you. What you do to better yourself will only reflect positively on those who love you. I am so excited for more of you to become enlightened by Jill's wisdom, just as I have been.

Jennifer Erickson
THIN CHOICES participant

THIN CHOICES TESTIMONIALS

Written by participants in the *THIN CHOICES* Program and collected in class surveys and follow-up correspondence.

The most important thing that I learned is that thin people generally aren't thin because they're "lucky" and I am not overweight because I'm "unlucky." It's all about choices— educated choices.

— Leanne S.

Being thin and healthy doesn't mean being deprived of the "good" things.

—Julie S.

I will never forget Jill. She changed my life. After attending her classes I got pregnant. I only gained 35 pounds with this pregnancy, as opposed to the 70 pounds that I gained with my first child. I very quickly returned to my pre-pregnancy weight and lost an additional 10 pounds to reach my ultimate goal weight. I will never yo-yo diet again.

—Jamie O.

I wish I had met Jill and discovered the THIN CHOICES *concept 10 years ago. I could have saved the thousands of dollars that I have wasted on diet programs, prepackaged meals, diet pills, and club memberships.*

—Nancy M.

My cholesterol level was up over 200. After adopting the THIN CHOICES *program, my cholesterol dropped to 123!*

—Ben G.

Jill sure enjoys what she does. She helps people believe in themselves again. She has a definite gift.

—Angie H.

I was skeptical about another diet plan because I've tried them all. This approach is definitely different—not a diet at all—and it works.

—Joan K.

I can't believe how easy this is! I don't even feel like I am on a diet, just making a few changes, yet I am still losing weight.

—Richard M.

The THIN CHOICES *concepts are simple and make sense. We should do what thin people are doing if we want to look like them.*

—Bev O.

I now eat and move like my thin friends. For the first time in my life, I actually try on clothes when I am shopping. I used to just buy the biggest size, take it home to try it on, and pray that it would fit. What a gift it is to be able to shop in the same clothing stores as everyone else.

— Janice K.

I will never go on another diet again. This non-diet approach has finally taught me how to lose weight without torturing my body. I have a new respect for this marvelous machine that serves me so well.

—Jennifer S.

My energy level is through the roof...without caffeine or drugs.

—Kenny R.

Since I have slowed down my eating pace, I really taste my food. I never knew that my wife was such a good cook!

—Ed D.

When Jill recommended that I should eat at least 8 to 10 servings of fruit and vegetables, I thought she was crazy! I wasn't eating any at that time. Now, 30 pounds lighter, I crave fruit and veggies daily. The bonus is that I am decreasing my risk of cancer at the same time.

—Anne F.

I now know that I am the one who made myself fat, and I am the only one who can make myself thin again. It is up to me; no one else can do it for me. I am through making excuses for my extra fat and done feeling sorry for myself.

—Jean F.

I didn't realize that I was slowly killing myself with the things I was putting into my body combined with my lack of activity. My weight was steadily increasing each year. After just one year of following the THIN CHOICES program, I feel great! I feel strong and lean. It is as if I have taken years off of my life. I have transformed from a tired slug into a beautiful butterfly.

—Amy B.

INTRODUCTION

When I was 16 years old, I was diagnosed with several food allergies. I began reading food labels to determine which foods contained the ingredients, preservatives, or colorings that would cause a negative reaction. I became fascinated with the science of nutrition and how the body is fueled by food. It seemed a natural decision to study nutrition in college.

Over the course of six years, I completed a bachelor of science degree in dietetics and a master's degree in nutritional sciences...and gained a total of 40 pounds! Ironically, I knew that I wanted to work with overweight people, helping them to lose weight. I blamed the fad of stretch pants and big, baggy sweaters for allowing me to gain weight without being aware. I did, of course, ignore the fact that I could no longer wear any of my blue jeans.

When I finally admitted that I was overweight, I began to take a closer look at my eating and exercise (or lack of) habits. I had always lived within three blocks of the college campus. My goal was to sleep late and yet get to class in less than five minutes. I never ate breakfast, ate out at least two times each day, and often ate after midnight. I rarely drank water, but I could easily drink 8 to 12 cans of diet soda in a day. The only fruit or vegetables I consumed came mixed in the ice cream flurry or on the Subway foot-long sandwich.

I decided that I either needed to make some major changes in my lifestyle or resign myself to the fact that I would never be a credible source of nutrition information for anyone. My first self-imposed challenge was to move 2 miles away from campus. I then purchased a bicycle for transportation. My second challenge was to resist the urge to eat after midnight. I didn't set my goals too high, because I wanted to be sure to succeed in these first small steps. I quickly remembered how much I loved bicycling and started riding just for fun in addition to cycling to and from classes. Not eating after midnight was harder at first, but I finally adapted.

I then replaced the diet soda with water. I suffered a throbbing headache for three days, but again, my body adapted. I found that the more water that I drank, the thirstier I became. I began to enjoy and crave water. I was then ready to add fruit and vegetables to my diet. This was difficult, because I only liked bananas and mushrooms. I started with these two items and expanded my choices a bit at a time.

Gradually, I began to cut back on the junk food and excess fat in my diet, which was difficult because I didn't know how to cook anything more exotic than homemade macaroni and cheese, loaded with Velveeta. I taught myself how to cook using low-fat food choices and healthy cooking methods. I would cook, taste, revise, and record the changes that needed to be made the next time I made each recipe. Over a period of years, my collection of recipes became enormous. It was overflowing with great tasting, low-fat foods and beverages that tasted great and were good for me!

When I started my first job as a registered dietitian, 25 pounds lighter, the administrator of the hospital asked me to teach a weight-loss class for the community. I sent away for information about four existing weight-loss programs that I could purchase to teach the class. Each program contained some element that I thought would either make it too complicated for the participants or would seem too much like a restrictive diet. I decided to design my own program using my nutrition knowledge and personal experience. The participants were successful in losing weight and in keeping it off, something none of the programs I originally considered could claim. I knew I'd found my calling.

I went on to design a weight-loss program for two different hospitals and a fitness center in my community, continuing to teach my weight-loss techniques over the course of the next 10 years. During my many years of teaching, I learned what worked and what didn't, drawing on my experiences with clients and casually observing the habits of thin people. Whether the thin people I observed had always been thin or had lost weight and kept it off, they all seemed to be doing the same things—the same things that I was teaching in my classes. I then began formally interviewing thin people to dig deeper into their thought processes and practices to fine-tune my program.

I can help you learn how to live like a thin person by teaching you how to make a few simple changes in your lifestyle. These changes will be painless and quite an eye-opening experience. The choices that you make every day will ultimately determine what your body looks like and how you feel living in it.

Too many people are uncomfortable with their bodies. Life is too short to live in a body that you don't or can't enjoy. I want you to read this book, then begin to make a few simple changes, one at a time, in your eating and lifestyle habits. You will be amazed at how quickly your body responds.

Everyone knows what "thin" means to them. Although your weight-loss goal may be different than your spouse's or friend's, everyone will benefit from following the *THIN CHOICES* concepts. You will lose excess body fat, experience more energy, and increase your sense of well-being—all without feeling like you are on a restrictive diet.

My clients have been quite successful reaching their weight-loss goals over the last decade using the *THIN CHOICES* program. With this book, I hope to enlighten even more of you. This is not another diet plan with a restrictive menu that you follow and then fall off. Use the information in this book as a guideline for acquiring new habits that will last a lifetime.

Starting with my *THIN CHOICES* program as the foundation, I have added some of the most common habits of thin people. The people I observed are staying thin as a way of life.*

With this book, you have the knowledge of how to become and stay thin. You will never need to go on another diet or spend another dime of your hard-earned money on the latest weight loss fad or pill. Congratulations!

Everyone wants to know what thin people do to stay thin. Some of their best inspirational quotes are highlighted and interspersed throughout the chapters.

---

* The criteria used to classify individuals as "thin people" for this book include: weight within normal limits according to current medically accepted height/weight charts, absence of past or present eating disorders, and being a nonsmoker (nicotine is noted to raise metabolic rates).

CHAPTER 1

Thin People
Don't "Diet"

*Become thin for the rest of your life
without ever going on another "diet."*

Diets do not work!

The word *diet* is defined by Webster's dictionary as "what a person or animal usually eats and drinks; daily fare." The majority of people, however, hear the word *diet* and think of the more common meaning: "to deprive oneself of food to lose weight." For the purpose of this discussion, *diet* refers to such restrictive programs.

Restrictive diets do not work. Thin people know this simple fact and just don't do it. If diets worked, everyone would be thin. This is not the case, as two out of three Americans are either overweight or obese. People will tell you that their diet works when they follow it. The truth is that a diet does not work if you are not able to sustain, long-term, a healthy weight.

Statistics show that 98 percent of dieters regain their lost weight within three years of initially losing it. Most diets are not designed to help you alter your lifestyle; thus they are doomed to fail.

The weight-loss industry knows that you are vulnerable and willing to do whatever it takes, no matter what the cost, to become thin. You have been willing to take pills without understanding the chemicals that you are consuming, follow liquid diets for weeks, eat soup by the gallons, and go against everything you have ever learned about good nutrition by eating only cheeseburgers, bacon, and eggs all day. Although most Americans who aren't thin seem to be obsessed with becoming thin, we are a statistically overweight nation.

Why Diets Don't Work

When you are on a diet, you restrict your intake of calories and certain foods over a period of time. You feel hungry, but you choose not to eat. Your body perceives that it is starving, so instead of shedding excess fat, it hangs onto it. You cannot starve a fat cell. It is far too smart.

Your body's primary goal is to survive and it will do anything to keep you alive, despite your desire to be thin. Therefore, your metabolism, or basal metabolic rate (BMR), dramatically slows the rate at which it burns calories. In this situation, your weight loss consists primarily of water and lean muscle loss. When you go off of the diet, your body takes the extra calories coming in and stores them as fat, just in case you decide to try to starve it again.

Many of you have been on a diet, lost weight, and then regained all of the weight you lost plus several extra pounds. You believe that diets don't work; you are right. The information in this book is based on the scientific understanding of how your body processes food for energy and of how you can easily raise your metabolism with a few simple lifestyle changes.

Muscle vs. Fat

Pound for pound, muscle takes up less space under your skin than fat. Think about the volume of a 1-pound lean tenderloin steak in comparison to one pound of lard, which is 100 percent fat. The steak is much more condensed in size, yet weighs exactly the same as the lard on a scale. Which would you rather have lying under your skin and your clothes? The muscle, of course! So our goal is to keep the muscle.

Two people who are the same height can weigh exactly the same on a scale, yet one person can look much heavier than the other based on each person's total body fat. If one is quite active and lifts weights on a regular basis and the other is sedentary, the person with the active lifestyle will appear much thinner. See the two figures below.

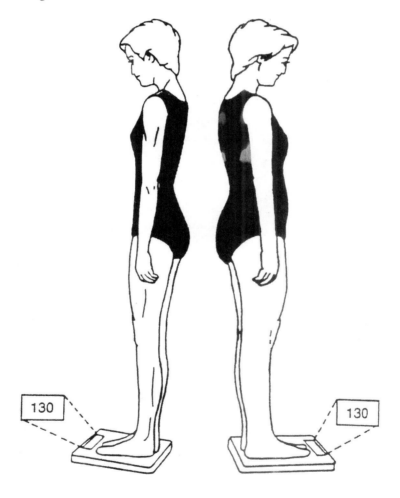

Most people with a desire to lose weight will look at these two ladies and say that they both look great or that it would be wonderful just to weigh 130 pounds, without regard to muscle. Try not to get hung-up on these images or weights. The purpose of showing these ladies is to illustrate the point that your number on a scale is not near as important as the actual composition of your body.

The person with the lower percentage of body fat will also be able to consume more calories than the sedentary one. This is because it takes more calories to sustain the lean muscle mass. Plus her jeans will fit much better! Which person would most of us rather be?

Muscle is metabolically active and actually burns calories. One pound of muscle can burn up to 45 calories per day. The more muscle we have, the higher our metabolism. Fat, on the other hand, is quite lazy and burns relatively few calories (less than 2 calories per pound per day). So to burn more calories, even while you are sleeping, your goal is to increase your lean muscle mass. This will get your body to start working for you. (See Chapter 12 for helpful information about increasing your lean muscle mass.)

Why Do You Keep Gaining Weight?

If your goal is to gain weight, then you should go on a diet, as this is the best way to increase your body weight and percentage of body fat. The ideal formula for weight gain is to go on a diet, lose 10 to 15 pounds, go off of the diet and gain 20 pounds, and then repeat the cycle. Does this sound familiar?

While on the subject of gaining weight, let's take a look at the two patterns of eating that can also help you gain weight. The first pattern (usually starting on Monday mornings) involves skipping breakfast, eating a lettuce salad with only vinegar or lemon juice for lunch, and then beginning to snack on large volumes of chips and cookies at approximately 3:00 P.M. Eating a large supper and an ice cream sundae shortly before going to bed would then finish off the day. Repeat this pattern several times each week for optimal weight gain.

The second pattern of eating that promotes weight gain is to follow a very strict, low-calorie diet from Monday morning until Friday early afternoon. Starting Friday afternoon, allow yourself a few extra treats and then go out for a high-fat, high-calorie supper. Continue to eat anything and everything that sounds tasty all through Sunday late into the evening. Then repeat this cycle the following week and you are sure to gain weight.

All joking aside, a lot of people believe that they have been following a weight-loss program, but have actually been gaining weight because the program was so restrictive they were either "on the diet" or "off the diet." This all-or-nothing mentality is one of the major factors influencing adult obesity. The "feast or famine" cycle of the past has evolved into the "diet or binge" cycle of today.

The All-or-Nothing Mentality

"Starting a new diet tomorrow" is the excuse given by people who exhibit the all-or-nothing mentality for eating too much food. Some of my weight-loss clients have admitted to consuming large quantities of food prior to starting a weight-loss program. One client said that she ate all of the chocolate in her house the day before starting her latest diet so she wouldn't be tempted by it while on the restrictive program. She truly believed that she was never going to eat chocolate again.

Another client stated that he needed to gain 15 pounds in order to be 100 pounds over his ideal weight so his insurance company would cover the expense of a weight-loss program. This is crazy!

By following a program that allows you to individualize your plan and requires you to eat meals and snacks fairly regularly, you will feel less deprived and be much more successful. You will be in control instead of allowing the cravings to control you. You will find that you are able to eat a small piece of chocolate instead of the whole box at one sitting.

Since this is a lifestyle change program and not a diet, you cannot fail. By the time you finish reading this book, you will have acquired too much information to ever totally go back to your old habits. You will learn to make good choices most of the time and not beat yourself up when you make the occasional poor choice. You don't want to be perfect, just better...and thinner.

As you now begin to observe thin people for yourself, you will notice that they do not have perfect diets and perfect exercise programs and perfect lives. It just seems that way because they look good in their blue jeans. Most thin people don't dwell on the negative aspect of their lifestyle choices. Instead of saying, "I blew it!" they might say, "I had a treat today." They turn a potentially negative situation into a positive one.

Lifestyle Change Program

The primary question you need to ask yourself when evaluating any new diet should be, "Can I follow this program for the rest of my life?" If your answer is "no," then do not even think about starting it. It will only cost you money and heartache when you are unable to continue with the unrealistic changes. You will feel like a failure, when it is the diet that has failed you.

Now that you know what thin people don't do, you need to begin to examine what they *are* doing to stay thin. The following chapters identify the strategies thin people use to control their weight and outline proven weight-loss techniques. These techniques are based on biochemical processes that occur within your body and have been used repeatedly—and successfully—in the *THIN CHOICES* program.

To find the perfect, permanent lifestyle change program that fits your needs, you will have to individualize the plan. This is easier than it may sound. Follow the majority of guidelines that are recommended in this book. The more of the guidelines you follow, the quicker you will begin to see your thin body start to emerge. Again, don't aim for perfection; focus on being "pretty good" most of the time. Instead of working against your body, you are going to learn how to listen to it and give it what it needs to enable you to achieve your optimal health and weight-loss goals. Do not give up your favorite foods but figure out how you can incorporate those desired choices into your plan. All foods can fit into this program. Your goal with the less healthy foods will be moderation not abstinence. You will also begin to notice that, as you follow the guidelines, your favorite food choices may begin to gradually change. Your body will begin to crave more of the foods that actually feed it, not just the ones that temporarily satisfy your mouth and mind.

Attitude

Your attitude will determine your success. You need to realize that you alone are responsible for your body and its size. Yes, you can continue to blame your mother for your saddlebags or your father for your apple-shaped abdomen, but what good does that do? You need to quit blaming others and start taking responsibility. Heredity definitely does play a role in predicting your body shape, but you alone are in charge of feeding it and moving it. How you choose to feed and move your body will ultimately determine your appearance.

Think positively and tell yourself you are doing a good job to stay motivated. Take on a partner who has similar weight-loss goals, so your friend can pep you up on a day that you are feeling discouraged and vice-versa. A friend can also be a motivating exercise partner.

This program will produce slow, yet steady weight loss. You will lose approximately 2 pounds per week. Those who have a greater amount of weight to lose will lose much faster, especially in the beginning, with 5- to 7-pound loss being reported by many participants weekly. Do not become discouraged that you are not losing weight as fast as you did on a previous, more restrictive diet. Remember that you regained most or all of that weight. Your goal is permanent weight loss through simple lifestyle choices. As you get closer to your goal weight, your body will be more stubborn about using its final excess fat reserves for energy. This makes losing that last 5 to 10 pounds much more difficult. Be patient and consistent. Your body will eventually respond with just a few tweaks in your lifestyle choices.

Monitoring Body Composition Changes

It is best to evaluate your body composition or weight changes using a clothing tape measure or a pair of fitted pants instead of solely relying on the scale. When you measure yourself, be sure to include your chest, waist, hips, buttocks, a thigh, and any other area that you would like to see less of. If you use a pair of pants or jeans as your measuring device, make sure you choose a smaller pair when the current pair is no longer snug enough to notice the subtle changes.

If you do choose to use a scale to evaluate your weight changes, it is best to weigh yourself at the same time of the day while wearing approximately the same amount of clothing. Weighing yourself once a week on the same day of the week will be the most consistent measure of your progress. Friday is often the best day since Monday weights can vary considerably because of inconsistencies in weekend habits. Early morning weights, prior to eating or drinking, tend to be the lowest and most consistent.

Weight variations can be subtle and will not always register accurately on the scale. Exercise can also cause a temporary weight gain according to the scale, because of a temporary fluid shift in the beginning due to muscles retaining water. After a week or so, this fluid readjusts and leaves the body.

Keep in mind that excess sodium from a meal one day may show up as water weight gain the next day. The bloated feeling that often accompanies the first few days of the menstrual cycle will also present as a temporary weight gain. It is best to avoid the scale on these days to help keep a positive attitude.

Visualization

Every night before going to sleep, close your eyes, take a deep breath, and visualize yourself at your goal weight. You may need to dig out some old pictures of yourself when you felt at your best. Picture yourself walking along the beach in a swimsuit. How do you look? How do you feel? Drown out the negative, self-defeating thoughts. Are you walking proud with your head held high? Are other people on the beach noticing how good you look?

For a small group of individuals, performing this visualization may seem scary. The thought of a swimsuit alone scares most people. During this visualization exercise, you may find that you feel anxious because you are no longer hiding behind your shell and people can actually see you. When you are covered by your fat suit, you blend in and it feels safe. If you have experienced these feelings, please be aware that losing weight is going to be a little intimidating in the beginning. It would be beneficial to anticipate and confront these issues now, because as a thin person, you will no longer be camouflaged.

This visualization process helps you prepare to start thinking like a thin person. Once you start eating and moving as a thin person would, it will be an easier transition if you also begin feeling and living like one at the same time. By feeling like a thin person feels, you will find that it is much easier to make healthy food choices, and you will actually find that your energy levels are higher. The mind is a powerful weight-loss tool.

Chapter 1:
Summary of Steps to Follow to Become a Thin Person

1. Resist the urge to ever go on another restrictive diet.

2. Find someone with weight-loss goals similar to yours as your weight-loss buddy.

3. Visualize yourself at your goal weight for five minutes every night before drifting off to sleep.

4. Begin thinking and feeling like the thin person that you will become.

CHAPTER 2

Thin People Eat Breakfast

Breakfast—the most important meal of the day

Why do I need to eat breakfast?

Thin people always eat breakfast because it is the most important meal of the day. As the word implies, breakfast is "breaking the fast." Unless you eat in the middle of the night, you fast throughout the night. Your metabolism, which is the rate at which your body burns calories, slows during this fasting period. By eating within an hour of when you wake, you break the fast, which tells your body to begin burning calories at a faster rate.

Visualize your metabolism as a campfire. To start a campfire, you start with a small amount of kindling. As the fire starts to burn, you add a little more wood, wait and then enjoy. If you continue to add a little wood, as it burns low, you can enjoy a steady fire all day long. This is very similar to how your metabolism works. If you add a little food in the morning and continue to add more food in small quantities all day long, you will have a steady "fire" burning calories all day long.

Just as you do not throw all of the wood in a pile to start a fire, you do not need a large amount of food to jump-start your metabolism either. Don't take this second step to mean that you need to eat an enormous breakfast. Rather, like the small amount of kindling needed to start the fire, only a small amount of food is needed to start your day out right.

No Excuses: Just Do It!

If you currently skip breakfast because you think you are too busy, have something that can be eaten quickly, such as a banana or a low-fat snack bar. Eating fast is not ideal as a general rule. But if you only have a minute or two in the morning, it is far better to eat something quickly instead of not at all. You can always eat that banana on your drive to work if you are really running late.

If you just can't tolerate any food in the early morning hours, start with something small, like a few crackers. You only need enough fuel to wake up your digestive system and get your body to begin burning calories. If you have a sensitive stomach in the morning, avoid eating fruit or drinking fruit juice on an empty stomach. These items may be too acidic for you.

If you think that coffee is the only fuel your body needs in the morning, think again. The caffeine in the coffee will not be effective in getting your metabolism started, and worse, it will fool your body into thinking that it is not hungry. Approximately 30 minutes after you've finished your last cup of java, you will be extremely hungry. Then you will find yourself looking for whatever is most readily available, often the high-fat doughnuts, cookies, or other bakery items that well-meaning coworkers provide.

In the previous scenario, you not only miss out on burning the extra calories that you would have if you had eaten breakfast, but you have also consumed enough fat and calories to smother your fire. (Avoiding the sugar/fat combination [and why bakery items are some of the worst "fat-storing" culprits] is discussed in Chapter 8.)

When is the best time to eat?

Ideally, you should eat something within the first hour of waking up. The sooner you eat something after waking up, the sooner you will begin to burn calories at a higher rate. If you forget to eat something within the first hour of waking up, eat something as soon as you do remember so that every waking hour can be a fat-burning hour.

Some people don't like to eat breakfast because they are then hungry all day long. This is a positive result of eating breakfast. It means that your body has used the food you've consumed and is ready for more. It means you are burning more calories.

One woman reported that she ate breakfast at 9:00 A.M. However, she was waking up at 5:00 A.M. Once she started eating just a handful of grapes at 5:00 A.M., she found that she was actually hungry and ready to eat her real breakfast at 7:00 A.M. and could no longer wait until 9:00 A.M. to eat. With the change she made, her body quickly burned the calories from the grapes, then sent her the message that more fuel/food was needed. Consequently, she began burning more calories all day long and began losing weight quickly and effortlessly.

The thin people who were surveyed all reported eating breakfast. The surprising finding was that most ate a very light breakfast meal. The majority ate a slice of toast or a small bowl of cereal. They also included a small glass of fruit juice or a serving of fruit.

Now you have the second step thin people follow. Forget the excuses for not eating your breakfast and just do it. Kick-starting your metabolism and burning calories at a higher rate all day is one of the best ways to get your body working for you.

Chapter 2:
Summary of Steps to Follow to Become a Thin Person

1. Eat something for breakfast within the first hour of waking up every day.

CHAPTER 3

Thin People Eat When They Are Hungry

By ignoring hunger, you miss the opportunity to burn calories.

Hunger Versus Desire

Thin people eat when they are hungry, which keeps their bodies burning calories efficiently. This rule assumes that you *know* when you are hungry. If you've been dieting for many years, you probably don't know how to tell when (or if) you are hungry. Webster's dictionary describes hunger as "the discomfort, pain, or weakness caused by a need for food." To think of hunger as the *need* for food helps keep the term fairly objective. We are talking about your body's need for fuel, not your mouth's desire for chocolate or potato chips.

Thin people often describe hunger as "feeling empty," or they may say, "My body needs fuel." The signals that indicate they are hungry include hunger pangs

> "I eat for energy."
>
> —Janet F.

and a growling stomach. Some thin people state that they if they become too hungry, they feel light-headed. (This could be related to low blood sugar.)

Thin people almost always eat because they are truly hungry, whereas overweight people tend to eat for a variety of other reasons. This is not to say that thin people never eat because of stress or to celebrate, but it is less likely for them to eat for these external reasons. Try to picture where your appetite is on the following hunger-satisfaction scale before you start eating.

Hunger-Satisfaction Scale (HSS)

10: Stuffed to the point of feeling sick (Thanksgiving full!)
9: Very uncomfortable, tired
8: Uncomfortably full
7: Feel you have eaten just a little bit too much
6: Comfortable, satisfied
5: Just noticing the first signs of hunger
4: Hungry, ready to eat
3: Very hungry
2: Extremely hungry, irritable
1: Starving, can't concentrate, dizzy

Ideally, you should eat when you notice that you are at a number four or five on this scale. You should be physically hungry when you begin each meal or snack. Don't eat just because the food is there. In a perfect world, your appetite would remain in the four to six range all of the time.

Thin people know that if they eat when they notice the first signs of hunger, they are better able to make healthy food choices and stay in control. Ignoring your hunger signals is missing the chance to burn calories. You may also feel out of control in your food choices if you wait until you feel like you are starving (one or two on the scale).

An overweight person often waits to eat until dropping to a two or one on the hunger-satisfaction scale. As a result, two things happen. First, you look for the easiest-access, highest-fat foods available. At a one or two, you aren't thinking clearly and don't care about fat, calories, or your health. Second, at a one or two, the tendency is to eat quickly to make the uncomfortable feeling go away, barely even tasting the food or taking the time to chew. This scenario often takes place in a person's car after pulling out of the fast food drive through.

Thin people do report similar experiences but go on to qualify that it doesn't happen often. By carrying healthy snacks with you (see Chapter 5), you are prepared for such a crisis and can take the time to find a better choice other than fast food for your next meal.

Getting in Touch With True Hunger

You may not yet be in touch with your hunger signals. Some overweight people don't even eat in relation to hunger, because they never get hungry. This may be because they consistently eat too large of portions of high-fat foods. If this sounds familiar, you will need to relearn the feeling of hunger. This will take practice. By decreasing the fat in your diet (Chapter 8) and eating fist-sized portions (Chapter 3), you will begin to experience hunger pangs approximately three or four hours following a meal and one or two hours after a small snack.

The fear of hunger is the hidden enemy of many people trying to lose weight. Ask yourself, "Is my body requesting food or is my mind just craving it?" A person who is truly hungry is willing to eat practically anything, even a food he or she may dislike. One thin person interviewed liked to ask herself, "Am I raisin hungry?" because she didn't particularly like raisins. This didn't mean that she ate raisins; rather she used the question as a guideline to determine if she was truly hungry.

Psychological Cravings

If you are only hungry for a specific food, you are most likely experiencing psychological hunger, or a craving. Cravings are often stimulated by food cues, such as smelling or seeing food. You may be watching television when a commercial for pizza appears, and it causes you want to eat pizza. Or you may finish a satisfying meal at a restaurant, and the waiter brings the dessert menu or cart to your table, causing you to want something sweet.

When dealing with cravings, the 20-minute distraction strategy is very useful. Find something to keep you occupied, or distracted, for 20 minutes until the craving passes. Ideally this activity will be something that involves both your brain and your body, such as rearranging the furniture or playing the piano. Nutrition researchers have found that after 20 minutes of ignoring mental hunger, or being distracted, the craving almost always subsides.

Emotional Eating and Alternative Activities

Mental hunger can also be triggered by your emotions. The urge to eat may be brought on by feelings of anxiety, depression, anger, frustration, boredom, loneliness, sadness, or even happiness. Some people who are lonely or bored find themselves eating without really thinking about what they are doing. They use food as a friend to keep them company and fill the voids.

If you currently eat for reasons other than true hunger, you first need to identify what those reasons are. The best way to do this is to carry a journal with you for a minimum of three consecutive days. One of these days should be a weekend day. In this journal, write down everything that you eat and list why you ate it. Did you eat the sandwich because it was lunch time or because you were hungry? Below is a sample page from an eating journal.

Day:	Time:	Food/beverage consumed	Why did I eat/drink it?
Mon.	7:00 a.m.	black coffee	caffeine
	7:50 a.m.	banana	to start my metabolism
	10:00 a.m.	2 slices toast with jam 2 eggs, over-easy	hungry
	12:00 p.m.	Big Mac & large French Fries, 16 oz. diet Coke	it was lunch time/ socializing/thirsty
	2:00 p.m.	Candy bar (full-sized)	tired
	4:00 p.m.	Water	thirsty
	5:00 p.m.	Chips with dip	hungry/making dinner
	6:00 p.m.	Lasagna, carrots & garlic bread	family was eating/not hungry
	8:00 p.m.	Ice Cream with Chocolate sauce	bored/not hungry

You will probably begin to notice your eating patterns quite quickly. You will be amazed to realize how many times you are eating throughout the day without even being hungry. Once you identify your personal eating triggers, make a list of alternative activities to do when any of these feelings arise.

For instance, if you usually eat when you are bored, make a list of 10 things you can do the next time that you are bored. For example, clean a closet, take five deep breaths, read a chapter in your book, take a bubble-bath, drink a glass of water, take a walk around the block, or call a friend. The next time you are feeling bored, choose one of the alternative activities on this list and do it. If you go for a walk, you experience the added benefit of burning calories instead of consuming them at a time when your body does not need the food. You'll be surprised how quickly you adapt to substituting your alternate activities for eating.

Take a few minutes right now to make an alternative activity list. Use the template shown below. List the 10 things you can do the next time you have a desire to eat for reasons other than true hunger. Use some of the suggestions listed above to get you started. Hang your list on the inside of the cupboard door you typically open when looking for food.

Instead of Eating I Could...

Make a list of activities other than eating that make you feel good. Refer to this list and choose one of these activities as alternatives to eating when you're not hungry.

1. _____

2. _____

3. _____

4. _____

5. _____

6. _____

7. _____

8. _____

9. _____

10. _____

Here is another useful tool that will help control your urge to eat for psychological or emotional reasons. It is called the Eating Triggers and Solutions worksheet. You can list the triggers that cause you to eat for reasons other than hunger, then list the solution. This completed worksheet should also be readily available to you and placed near your usual eating area.

Eating Trigers & Solutions Worksheet

Eating Triggers	Solutions
1. Anger	1. a. Talk to someone about it
	b. Take a bubble bath
	c. Hit a punching bag/pillow
2. Boredom	2. a. Clean a closet—keep busy
	b. Call a friend
	c. Get out of the house
3. Craving sweets	3. a. Eat a fruit (nature's sweets)
	b. Brush & floss teeth
	c. Chew gum
4. Tired	4. a. Take a nap
	b. Go to bed for the night
	c. Do some jumping jacks
5. Stress	5. a. Go for a 10 minute walk
	b. Take a hot shower
	c. Do some deep breathing

You can tailor this worksheet to match your own eating triggers and possible solutions according to your personality. The key is to plan ahead. Plan how to handle the situation or emotion before it occurs. Most deviations from your healthy eating program will occur on impulse, when you have no time to make rational choices.

Thinking logically, it makes sense to address your feelings rather than routinely using food to suppress them. When you think about it, it really is crazy that we eat because we are tired or sad. Take that nap or buy yourself flowers instead. With a little practice, you can learn to control emotional eating.

Digestion

Once you start eating breakfast, you will find that you become hungry sooner than you did before. How soon you become hungry depends on what and how much you eat for breakfast. If you eat a large breakfast with a lot of fat, like bacon and eggs with buttered toast or a couple of doughnuts, you won't be hungry for a long time. The fat, as well as the protein, takes longer to digest and will keep you feeling full longer, possibly as long as six or seven hours.

Carbohydrates, on the other hand, are relatively easy for the body to digest and use for fuel. So if you have a slice of toast with jelly and a banana, you will probably be hungry within two hours. The lighter breakfast is preferable if you know you will be able to eat again in a few hours. If you won't be able to eat a few hours later, add some protein or fat, such as an egg or some peanut butter to the lighter breakfast to stay satisfied a little longer.

Your stomach is approximately the same size as your fist. So make a fist and look at it. This is the how large your volume of food should be at a meal or a snack. Ideally you will be eating one to three fist-sized portions of food every three to four hours after a meal or every one to two hours after a snack. This guideline will help you if you aren't in touch with your hunger and satiety signals yet.

> "I eat many small meals a day and I work it off by keeping active."
>
> —Mary F.

Studies show that the ability to digest large volumes of food slows in women 50 and over. They are more likely to store the extra calories as fat. However, women in that age range continue to process calories just as efficiently as younger people when they are consumed in small amounts. This is yet another reason to eat small, frequent meals throughout the day.

Chapter 3:
Summary of Steps to Follow to Become a Thin Person

1. Ask yourself how hungry you are before you start eating a meal or a snack.

2. Eat if you are truly hungry, do something else if you are not.

3. Stop eating when you are satisfied or no longer hungry, not full.

4. Keep your hunger level between a four and a six on the HSS most of the time.

5. Complete the "Eating Triggers and Solutions" worksheets. Refer to it as needed.

6. Decrease the volume of food you eat to 1-3 fist-sized portions per feeding.

CHAPTER 4

Thin People Don't Clean Their Plates

Membership to the "clean plate club" comes with hidden costs.

Fuel Your Body, Not Your Soul

Why would you ever continue to pump gas into your car's gas tank once it is full? You wouldn't, because if you did, it would spray all over you. If your body sprayed all excess food back out, most people wouldn't feed it more than it requires. Fortunately for the embarrassment factor but unfortunately as far at weight control is concerned, our body won't reject what it doesn't need. It will accept the excess food and store it as fat.

As noted in Chapter 3, most thin people have learned how to listen to their body's need for food. They start eating when they begin to notice the first signs of hunger and stop eating once they are satiated. Looking back at the hunger-satisfaction scale, note where you are on the scale when you stop eating.

> "The three main reasons I stop eating are: I am satisfied, the food no longer tastes good, or some other activity needs to be completed."
>
> —Nikki K.

29

Ideally, you begin eating when you notice that your hunger level is at a number four or five on the scale. Most thin people stop at six (occasionally a seven). Thin people often comment that they would rather feel a little bit hungry than uncomfortably full. Overweight people often eat to an eight, nine, or even ten. When questioned as to why they routinely eat to that level, the response is the same: "The food just tasted so good!" or "This is a special occasion."

Slow Down and Really Taste Your Food

"The food just tasted so good" is the response given most often by overweight people. But by eating too fast, you don't even have the opportunity to taste your food. The enjoyment in eating happens in your mouth. If you really want to enjoy your food, learn to keep it in your mouth longer to really savor it. This practice is called the art of sensuous eating.

Experiment with one M&M candy. Close your eyes, take a deep breath and put the M&M into your mouth. Your goal is to see how long you can keep the M&M in your mouth without swallowing it. Most people will be astonished to find out that, when totally focusing on the taste of the food, they are able to make that one M&M last for close to two minutes.

It was once reported that Jackie Onassis loved sweets and tried up to three different desserts at a meal. Jackie's secret was that she would dip her fork into the cheesecake or other dessert, and then taste the small amount that stuck to the tines of the fork, savoring it in her mouth as long as she could. She would do the same with each dessert. As a result, she could enjoy the sensuous pleasure of tasting two or three different desserts without consuming all of the fat and calories that would accompany eating an entire one.

> "Eating slow keeps me from eating to the point of over-full."
>
> —Richelle J.

By slowing the pace at which you eat, you will learn to really enjoy the taste of your food. Thin people often comment that they love food and love to eat. The majority of thin people eat slowly with control and genuinely enjoy each bite. With this strategy, they are able to be more satisfied with less food. As discussed in Chapter 3, the reason that they are able to eat slowly is because they did not wait until they were famished to begin eating.

Another advantage of slower eating is that chewing your food thoroughly aids your body in digestion. The saliva in your mouth will begin to break your food down into pieces that are more manageable in size for your digestive tract to handle. Your body is able to absorb more of the vitamins and minerals from the food you eat when you chew them well. Have you ever noticed that a baby will sometimes have whole pieces of food in her diaper? This is because she has not yet learned how to chew her food well.

Sit Down and Focus

Many overweight people do a lot of "mindless eating." They eat while standing, preparing a meal, driving, reading, or watching television. If you find it difficult to either prepare a meal or clean up after a meal without tasting the food, chew a piece of gum to occupy your mouth so you cannot eat.

Choose a dining area and only eat while sitting in this area. At home your dining area may be the kitchen table, whereas at work your dining area may be the break room. This will take practice and time, but it will help you become much more aware of your food consumption.

Turn off the television and close the magazine. By only eating while you are eating, you will be able to focus your attention on what and how much you are eating. This will help in your effort to slow down, decrease your portion sizes, and listen for your body to give you the signal that it is satisfied.

Special Occasions Galore

The second excuse many overweight people give for eating too much is, "This is a special occasion." If you give yourself permission to overeat on every special occasion, you are overeating too often. With holidays, birthdays, weddings, parties, funerals, vacations, and even weekends considered "special occasions," you may be overeating several times each week.

Look back at your calendar over the last three months. How many "special occasions" can you count? Are you still considering each weekend as an opportunity to be more relaxed in what and how much you eat? It is not to say that you can't eat a piece of wedding cake. The guideline is that you should not eat the cake if you are already feeling uncomfortable from the foods you've already eaten.

Holidays

Try to build as much consistency into your holidays as possible. When you know that you have a holiday gathering to attend, stick to your usual routine as much as you can. First, wake up, exercise, and eat breakfast. Second, eat a snack to take the edge off your appetite before going to a family gathering or party. This will put you in control and make it easier to pass on the chips and appetizers. Third, bring a healthy dish to share. Fourth, stop eating when you are no longer hungry. Finally, remove or excuse yourself from the dining area to engage in some other form of entertainment.

This is in contrast to the way my family previously conducted their holiday meals. My whole family would engage in the huge festive meal. We all skipped breakfast to "save room" for the feast. We would start snacking on the pickles and M&Ms hours before the actual meal. After eating second and sometimes third servings of the feast, the majority of the males would excuse themselves to play cards, watch a ball game on television, or take a nap.

My grandma, aunts, and cousins would all continue to sit around Grandma's huge dining room table talking. The dishes would all be cleared away. Everything was removed except for the fork that each person kept in case there was more to eat. Then came the desserts. At this point, everyone remaining at the table would complain that they were feeling quite full.

Yet, as the desserts were passed, everyone sampled each one— just a fork-full of the pumpkin pie as the plate floated by, but eventually, each dessert plate was empty. Typically, after desserts, the debate over which diet to go on "once the holidays are over" began. (They were all planning on eating like this until the first of January!)

Now I poke fun of this crazy little holiday eating club of my family's, but I also belonged for years without seeing its dysfunction for what it was. I too held onto my fork and waited for my turn to stab the next whipped cream–covered dessert that passed my direction. My abdomen would be so bloated and full that my pants would be discreetly unbuttoned beneath my oversized sweater.

With all of the blood that would normally be pumping to my brain being redirected to my belly to help the food overload emergency, I couldn't keep focus on any of the conversations. Lucky for me, no one else was contributing anything too thought-provoking by this point. Although none of us had consumed a drop of alcohol, we all began to grow tired and slightly light-headed.

But one year, I stepped away from the table after only eating up to the "second helping" phase of the meal. Returning to the dining room an hour later, it seemed as if my family members had been deprived of oxygen in my absence. They were all lethargic— some of them were actually starting to nod off.

I couldn't believe what I was seeing. I was in awe. I couldn't understand why they were doing this to themselves. Didn't they realize that they were actually torturing themselves? From that day forward, I vowed to never punish my own body with holiday food again.

Pay Attention to Your Light Switch

Thin people are more likely to eat as a result of physical signals that indicate their bodies require food. Overweight people eat more often because of external signals, such as being in a social setting or being surrounded by good-tasting food. Once you become good at identifying your hunger and satiety, you too can eat like a thin person. You will be able to tell from one bite to the next when to stop eating.

"Going for a walk every holiday morning is a 'must' for me. It helps me make better food choices at the party and minimizes the stress that often accompanies the holidays."

—Natalie H.

Here is the trick. Once you have learned to tell how hungry and satisfied your body is, you will be eating slowly with control and chewing thoroughly. Then, almost as if a light switch being flipped, you will notice when you move to the next level on the hunger-satisfaction scale and are no longer hungry. What should you do? There is still food on your plate.

If you are eating like a thin person, you will stop eating. If you are eating like an overweight person, you will clean your plate (and probably order dessert too, since you have already blown it). Again, this is the all-or-nothing type of thinking you are now avoiding. Realize that it is all right to leave food on your plate. Give yourself permission to not eat it. See the breaking the chain model (page 35) for additional insight on how to deal with this scenario.

Breaking the Chain

We all have behavior chains that lead us to eat when we are not hungry or to overeat. The key to breaking your chain is to first identify the problem. You may have more than one bad be-havior chain that needs attention. Focus on the chain that causes you to overeat most often first and work on the others later.

If you are a member of the "clean plate club," your behavior chain may look something like this:

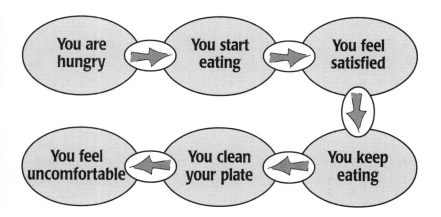

Your behavior chain is only as strong as its weakest link. Once you break one of the links, the whole chain is broken. The chain above needs to be broken after the "you feel satisfied" link.

What to Do with the Excess

People who have a difficult time stopping until their plate is clean usually have guilt associated with wasting food. Many of us can still hear our mother's voice telling us to be grateful and clean our plates because there are so many starving children in the world. We also remember that if we were "good" and cleaned our plates, we were then rewarded with something special or even dessert! Some of us just can't handle the guilt of throwing perfectly good food away. If this sounds familiar, you need to learn how to deal with this guilt.

What you decide to do with the food that is left on your plate is up to you. Here are a few suggestions provided by several thin people, as well as previous members of the clean plate club.

- Wrap up the leftover food to eat later. This will prevent any guilt from wasting the food, as you do plan to eat it later. Whether you actually eat this food later (or not) is not a concern when you wrap it up.

- Set a large glass jar on your counter. When you have eaten to the point of satisfied, dump the excess food into the jar. This visual reminder of how much excess food you have been eating (beyond what your body actually needs) will be astonishing. The excess food in this jar will also grow much faster if you normally eat your children's leftovers, too.

- Take the glass jar (above) or an ice cream bucket and when it is full of excess food, dump it into the garden for wonderful compost that will help your flowers and vegetables grow.

- Leave the excess food on your plate and cover it with a napkin. The food will no longer be a temptation. This works particularly well at a restaurant or a social function. The napkin over your plate signifies to the waiter that you are finished with your meal.

- Throw your excess food away and then send money to a charity that helps children who are starving. This will help ease your guilt over disposing of your excess food, plus children who are in need of food will benefit from your gesture.

You can try the old trick of using a smaller plate or just taking smaller portions in the first place to avoid large amounts of waste. But you still need to practice leaving food on your plate. If you don't practice this new habit, you will continue to eat to the point of being uncomfortable in situations where you have put too much food on your plate.

Picture your body storing fat in its fat cells every time you eat beyond the point of being satisfied. This is especially true when you eat to the point of feeling stuffed ("Thanksgiving full"). You are eating more food than your body needs to function and the excess has nowhere else to go, so it is stored as body fat. Start practicing with your next meal. Leave just a few bites on your plate and see how you feel. Do you feel guilty? Do you feel compelled to pick your fork back up? Take a few deep breaths and decide what to do with the excess food. This exercise will become easier every time that you do it. Pretty soon you will find that you are no longer a member of the clean plate club. Congratulations!

> "I do clean my plate as I do not like to waste food, so I typically only dish out a portion that I think would be adequate for a normal person and I don't go back for second helpings."
> —Paula D.

Breaking the Cycle

Once you break the behavior chain, also resolve to break the cycle. Avoid teaching your children and grandchildren to eat to the point of being uncomfortable. Do not use food as a reward for good behavior or to encourage kids to eat the "healthy" foods first.

All children are born with a natural sense of hunger and satiety. They request food when they are hungry and refuse food once that hunger has been satisfied. Observe a baby or a toddler to refresh your memory. It is only in our later years that we are taught to eat until we feel uncomfortable. As children, many of us were often rewarded for cleaning our plate with a trip to the zoo or an ice cream cone.

To recap, many overweight people are so used to feeling "stuffed," that they don't feel they should stop eating until they reach that state. If you have lost your natural desire to eat when you are hungry and to stop eating once your body has been satisfied, you need to relearn this skill. It will take some practice and will initially seem foreign to stop eating when you are no longer hungry, but eventually it will become second nature once again.

Chapter 4:
Summary of Steps to Follow to Become a Thin Person

1. Eat all food slowly, chewing well.

2. Pay close attention to what your body is saying to you.

3. Leave some food on your plate at one meal every day.

4. Do not give yourself permission to overeat, even on special occasions.

CHAPTER 5

Thin People Carry Snacks

You need to eat, and eat often, to lose weight and stay thin.

Is Your Gas Tank Running On Empty?

Picture your car's gas tank. Going too long without fueling your car causes it to run out of gas and stop working. Most of us don't like to risk an empty tank in the middle of the road, so we refuel when the gauge approaches the red "E." Your body is similar in its need for fuel (food). It doesn't operate well without a sufficient supply.

In Chapter 3 we discussed that thin people eat when they start to notice the first signals of hunger rather than waiting until they are famished. Thin people know that hunger can strike at any time, anywhere, and they are usually prepared to deal with their hunger. They prepare by carrying snacks and having them in their desk at work, in their car, in their purse, and even in their locker at the gym.

If it seems like your thin friends or coworkers are always eating, it is because they are. They are not embarrassed if they feel the need to eat a handful of nuts while they work on a project at their desk. Or you may notice them eating half of their sandwich that was meant for lunch, even though it is only 9:00 in the morning. If their bodies are sending hunger signals, thin people are usually responding to them with the additional fuel that is needed.

Thin people like to stash or carry their own snacks so they are prepared whenever and wherever hunger may strike. If they are caught in an unexpected traffic jam and will be 45 minutes late getting home for supper, they can have a little snack in the car so the Golden Arches

> "I like strong mints to take the edge off of my hunger in between meals."
>
> —Suzanne N.

won't tempt them as they pass through town. They know that without a snack, they will be so hungry by the time they get home they will dive into the bag of chips like a crazed animal.

> "I need to carry snacks—usually granola bars—because I get hungry between meals."
>
> —Amy M.

Have you ever noticed that thin people may just take a few bites of something and then put it away for later? They seem to have the utmost control, and we all envy them. They reason that they have such control is that they never let their body's fuel tank drop to the red "E"—ever! They are constantly functioning with their fuel tanks at least 1/8 to 1/4 full. Because they know that if they let their body approach the red "E," they are just as vulnerable to eating binges and junk food as the rest of us.

Chapter 5:
Summary of Steps to Follow to Become a Thin Person

1. Carry healthy snacks with you.
2. Eat a snack if you feel you are truly hungry.

Thin People Don't Go to Bed Full

Feeling full at bedtime will keep your fat cells plump and happy.

Hibernating bears don't need food.

When you are sleeping, your body's metabolism slows down significantly. You do not need food in your stomach to make it through the night. Think about a hibernating bear making it through the whole winter without eating. During hibernation, much like nighttime rest, caloric needs are drastically reduced and the body lives on fat reserves.

Most thin people stop eating at least two to three hours before going to bed. This gives their body enough time to digest the food they've consumed before lying down. Since weight loss is your goal, you may want to increase this amount of time to at least three hours. You may find it helpful to give yourself a cutoff time for your eating. For example, if you normally go to bed at 10:00 P.M., tell yourself that you will not eat or drink anything other than water after 7:00 P.M.

> "I don't eat anything after supper."
> —Jenny M.

When surveying thin people of all age ranges, they all described their hunger level at bedtime as somewhere between neutral and slightly hungry. Most of the thin people explained that they felt uncomfortable if they went to bed with a full stomach.

41

Where do my late-night-eating calories go?

If you go to bed feeling full, picture your body storing the extra calories as body fat. Visualize the chips and dip or ice cream with chocolate sauce floating directly into your fat cells. This is pretty close to reality. Because your metabolism is at its slowest while you are sleeping, your body does not need the extra calories for fuel. Instead, it will store the extra calories as fat in your fat cells.

When you go to bed feeling slightly hungry, the opposite happens. Your body pulls fat from its fat stores to use for the small caloric needs that it has at night. Your body is now working for you and even burning fat calories while you sleep.

Tricks to Prevent Late-Night Eating

If you find that you are having a hard time ignoring your hunger at bedtime, try brushing and flossing your teeth a little earlier than usual. You may also want to go to bed an hour or so before your usual bedtime to help your body learn to adjust to this change. Eventually, going to sleep while feeling somewhere between neutral and hungry will start to feel natural and you will be mobilizing stored fat throughout the night.

Researchers have found that television viewing is directly linked to snacking. Therefore, it would be beneficial to avoid watching television during the two or three hours prior to going to sleep. You may find that a good book or a relaxing bubble bath will help keep your mind elsewhere. If you have a favorite program that you don't want to miss, tape it and watch it in the morning during your exercise session. How is that for the perfect weight-loss scenario?

Chapter 6:
Summary of Steps to Follow to Become a Thin Person

1. Stop eating three hours before going to bed.
2. Choose a cut-off time for eating each day and don't eat or drink after that time.

CHAPTER 7

Thin People Eat Fruit and Vegetables

Something so simple as eating more fruit and vegetables vastly improves your health and decreases your waistline.

"Five-a-Day" for Better Health

You may remember hearing about the "five-a-day" campaign to increase the consumption of fruit and vegetables by Americans to a total of five servings per day. The American Cancer Society realizes the importance of a low-fat, high-fiber, anti-oxidant-rich diet in the prevention of cancer. As previously mentioned, a low-fat diet is also beneficial in promoting weight loss.

The majority of thin people surveyed all consumed between four and eight combined servings of fruit and vegetables every day. While you work to lose weight, it will benefit you to increase your intake to 8 to 10 servings per day. These foods have very few calories, are high in fiber,

> "I do not follow a special diet. I just really try to make sure to incorporate fruits and vegetables into every meal and leave out the fattening items."
>
> —Denise M.

and most are totally fat free, which makes them the perfect weight-loss food.

It may seem like a lot of fruit and vegetable servings at first, but with a little planning, it is a simple goal to achieve. Increasing your intake of fruit and vegetables will also help decrease the available room in your stomach for higher fat, less healthy foods.

Imagine a fruit bowl that contains a total of 10 servings of fruit and vegetables. Although the volume of food appears large, the total number of calories will only be an average of 410 calories, depending on which choices were made. This is fewer calories than you would find in your deli muffin or just one donut.

> "It's not only about what you are eating but also about what might be missing from your diet that is influencing your health and weight. Eating more fruit and vegetables automatically improves my whole diet."
>
> —Colin T.

Smoothies

An easy way to incorporate more fruits and vegetables into your diet is to drink smoothies. A smoothie is a blender drink that usually has either a milk, soymilk, yogurt, or fruit juice base with fresh or frozen fruits added. You can easily add three to five fruits to your smoothie and maybe even a vegetable. By drinking just one smoothie each day, you will meet half of your fruit and vegetable goal for the day.

When you first start making smoothies, limit the number of ingredients to three or four. A beginner's smoothie might be 1 cup of skim milk, 1 frozen banana (best if peeled prior to freezing), and 2 tablespoons of orange juice concentrate. Some people may find that adding a few ice cubes helps keep the smoothie cold. Blend this mixture until smooth and enjoy.

As you become more adventurous with your smoothies, you may find that adding a handful of frozen berries adds a nice zing.

A couple of baby carrots will add a little color, a bit of sweetness, and a few vitamins (antioxidants). A couple of tablespoons of flaxseed or wheat germ will add some texture and more healthy vitamins (vitamin E). Don't turn your nose up at any of these suggestions until you try them.

> "Drinking a smoothie every day makes it easy to get my fruit in."
> —Jen E.

Salads and the "Dipping Technique"

Choosing a salad for one meal each day will also help to substantially increase your vegetable consumption. You can load the salad up with vegetables and lean proteins. Be sure to have your salad dressing on the side. The dipping technique will start to become second nature to you. Dip the tines of your fork into the salad dressing (don't scoop), and then poke your fork into the salad. You will have salad dressing on every bite while only using a fraction of the dressing.

The dipping technique will help you learn to enjoy the taste of your vegetables again. They will not be drowning in dressing, which adds a lot of fat and calories. Studies have shown that most women get the majority of their fat intake from salad dressings and creamy sauces, which is why women in particular need to be very aware of how much dressing they are using.

You may prefer to choose low-fat or nonfat salad dressings, but this won't help you learn a new, healthier habit. The problem with buying fat free is that the next time you go to a restaurant or a friend's house where they only have regular-fat salad dressings; you will still be craving a large amount and will consume far too much fat. Try the dipping technique with your next salad. If you feel deprived, you can always add a little more at a time.

Drinking your fruit and vegetables

Drinking vegetable or tomato juice does count toward your intake of vegetables. By drinking one 12-ounce can of vegetable juice, you will have consumed the equivalent of three vegetables. However, the extra sodium in vegetable juice can cause your body to retain fluids. To prevent this, make sure that you are drinking extra water on the days that you drink vegetable juice.

Drinking fruit juice also counts toward your consumption of fruit, but the calories are very concentrated in fruit juices and excess calories can lead to weight gain. Think about how many oranges you have to squeeze to produce a glass of juice. It makes sense that a 12-ounce glass of orange juice contains 180 calories, whereas an orange only has 60. Limit your intake of fruit juice to less than 1 cup per day.

The calories from dried fruit also add up relatively quickly. Check the ingredient list to be sure that your banana chips weren't dipped in butter prior to being dehydrated. Portion size is very important when evaluating dried fruit. For example, one serving of raisins is only 2 tablespoons. Read the nutrition label to find the appropriate serving size.

Start Slowly

You may not like all fruit and all vegetables. But there are so many choices in these two food categories that there must be at least a few that you can tolerate. Start eating the few that you do like and then add a few new choices every week. The more fruit and vegetables you eat, the more your body will begin to crave them.

Begin increasing your intake of fruit and vegetables slowly, because with the extra fiber in these foods, you may experience some bloating and flatulence. Start by eating three servings total per day and add another serving every few days. As your body begins to adjust to the extra fiber in your diet, the bloating and flatulence will subside.

You may notice that your bowel movements start to float (in the toilet). This happens because of the increase in fiber and decrease in fat in your diet. This is normal and desirable.

Chapter 7:
Summary of Steps to Follow to Become a Thin Person

1. Eat 8 to 10 servings of fruit and vegetables every day. Eating just one smoothie and one large salad each day will accomplish this goal.

2. Experiment with smoothies to find a combination you like.

3. Use the dipping technique for salad dressings and sauces with all sauces served on the side.

CHAPTER 8

Thin People Limit Their Intake of Fat

Those who succeed at permanent weight loss limit fat.

Why Limit Fat?

You may have heard that you need to decrease your intake of fat to lose weight. Do you know *why* decreasing your fat intake will promote weight loss? Why would you adhere to a rule that you don't understand? Let's discuss the two main reasons for following a low-fat diet.

The first reason is that fat is more dense in calories than either protein or carbohydrates. Fat contains 9 calories per gram, whereas both protein and carbohydrates only contain 4 calories per gram. This means that you can eat twice the volume of protein or carbohydrates for the same number of calories. Calories do count. If you consume more calories than your body needs and uses, you will gain weight.

The second reason to follow a low-fat diet is that it takes fewer calories to digest fat than it does to digest either protein or carbohydrates. Fat is practically already in its storage form. You burn approximately 25 percent of the calories consumed just by digesting either protein or carbohydrate calories. Only 3 percent of fat calories are burned during the process of digestion.

This means that if you eat one large, 100-calorie banana, you will only have 75 of those calories available for potential fat storage. Whereas if you eat two slices of bacon, also approximately 100 calories, 97 of those calories will be available for potential fat storage. The caloric difference is significant and can mean the difference between losing and gaining weight.

It's all about Choices...*THIN CHOICES*

The national registry for those who have been successful in maintaining weight loss has concluded that the majority of individuals follow a high-carbohydrate, low-fat diet. Most of their diets contain less than 30 percent of calories from fat. This means that a diet that contains 1,500 calories would contain no more than 50 grams of fat. After years of working with weight-loss clients, I've found that women are quite content, yet highly successful at weight loss, limiting their intake of fat to a range of 30 to 40 grams per day and men to a range of 40 to 50 grams per day.

It's all about choices. You choose how you want to consume your fat grams each day. If you choose bacon and eggs for breakfast, you can put jelly on your toast instead of butter and skip the hash browns. If you would rather eat the hash browns, then skip the bacon. If you eat all of the high-fat choices at this meal and use up all of your allowed fat grams, plan to feel quite limited in your options the rest of the day, eating mainly fruit and vegetables.

Anita O., seeking to lose 20 pounds, said that she was not willing to give up her butter. She wasn't even willing to switch to whipped butter or a tub margarine to save fat grams. After two days following the *THIN CHOICES* program, she found that she much preferred one slice of cheese on her burger than a pat of butter on the bun. At this point, Anita has almost given up her added-fats habit all together and has reached her goal weight.

Counting Fat Grams

You may find that it is initially difficult to figure out how much fat you are consuming. The *THIN CHOICES* fat revealer guide (available at www.ThinChoices.com) can help you estimate the number of fat grams in your favorite foods, particularly combination dishes and restaurant meals.

The easiest way to figure out how much fat is in the foods that you eat is by looking at the labels. First look at the portion size and then at the number of total fat grams that the food contains. Be sure to multiply the number of fat grams by the number of portions that you consume. If one half cup of angel hair pasta has one gram of fat, but you eat 2 cups, then you must count four half-cup servings or 4 grams of fat.

Combination Dishes

For combination dishes, calculate all of the fat that is going into your recipe by multiplying the total fat grams by the number of servings that you are putting into the dish. For example:

Chicken Lasagna:	fat grams
4 (4-ounce) chicken breasts	16 oz x 1g fat per oz = 16 g
1 pkg lasagna noodles (8 servings)	8 svg x 1 g fat per svg = 8 g
24 oz jar of spaghetti sauce	6 svg x 3 g fat per svg = 18 g
16 oz container of nonfat cottage cheese	0 grams of fat
1 onion	0 grams of fat
1 pound spinach	0 grams of fat
16 ounces mozzarella cheese	16 oz x 4g fat per oz = 64 g
Spices and seasonings	0 grams of fat
Total =	106 grams of fat

To figure out the amount of fat per serving, divide by the number of servings your recipe makes. In the example above, divide 106 grams of fat by 12 servings to arrive at 8.8, or rounding up, 9 grams of fat. Each serving of lasagna contains 9 grams of fat.

Nine grams of fat in an entree is not very much at all. If you want your lasagna to be even lower in fat, you can decrease the amount of cheese that you put into your recipe. A little trick that works well with pasta dishes is to move all of the hard cheese to the top of the dish. Your entree still looks luscious, but the total amount of cheese in the recipe can be cut by at least half. The cottage cheese, in the middle layers, takes up the space that was previously occupied by the hard cheese.

It seems like you are doing a lot of counting at first, but most people eat the same 8 to 10 entrees over and over. Once you have figured out how much fat is in one portion of your favorite lasagna, chili, and stroganoff recipes, you will never have to figure it out again. Just be sure to keep a running list of all of your favorite recipes and their fat gram content.

Divide Your Fat Grams

An easy way to avoid consuming too much fat is to break your day up into the number of meals and snacks that you have daily. If you normally eat three meals and two snacks each day, with a fat gram allowance of 40 grams, allow yourself 15 grams of fat for both lunch and supper. This allows you a total of 10 grams for breakfast and your snacks. This strategy also helps you avoid reaching the end of the day without taking in enough fat, which can make you extremely hungry and more susceptible to eating binges.

Your body does require a minimum of 15 grams of fat every day to function properly. This fat is used to lubricate your organs and keep your skin soft and your hair looking shiny. If you are cutting your fat intake too low, you will begin to notice dry skin and hair.

By keeping track of the foods you eat as well as the fat grams they contain, you will begin to see where the fat is in your diet. Then you can eliminate the fats that you are willing to live without and decrease the portion size of those that you are not. The best method for monitoring your total daily intake of fat is to use a lifestyle diary. Find one that includes ample space for tracking your fruit and vegetable intake as well. A notebook will be just fine to get you started.

By using the *THIN CHOICES* lifestyle diary (available at www.ThinChoices.com), Annie K. found that the majority of fat in her diet came from the same 10 food sources. This helped make her fat gram counting quite easy. She simply memorized the fat gram content of each of these foods so that she wouldn't have to read the label or look it up every time that she ate one of these foods.

Don't Forget about the Protein

Be sure to consume enough protein. Since protein and fat are often found together, you need to be aware of whether or not you are reaching your protein intake requirement. Protein intake is necessary for muscle repair. It also helps to keep your appetite under control, preventing hunger cravings, since it delays the rate at which your stomach empties.

Consuming protein will help keep you alert. This is especially important to remember if you have an important project to work on or a meeting in the afternoon, when most people tend to get tired. Include some protein with your lunch meal for optimal alertness.

Women should consume an average of 6 ounces of protein per day. Each ounce of meat contains 7 grams of protein, so if you are reading labels, your goal should be to consume at least 42 grams of protein per day.

Men should consume an average of 6 to 9 ounces of protein per day. This translates to 42 to 63 grams of protein per day.

Ideally your intake of protein will come from lean protein sources, such as fish, poultry, lean meats, eggs, low-fat dairy, and soy products.

Fat Gram Counting Conquered

You don't need to count fat grams forever. Once you become good at counting fat grams and revising your recipes, you can lighten up. You will most likely decrease your consumption of fat just by monitoring and recording the fat found in your favorite foods. You will begin to make different and healthier choices based on your newfound knowledge.

You only need to return to counting fat grams and recording your food intake in a lifestyle diary if you fall back into your old eating patterns—those that caused you to gain weight in the first place. If that happens, you should focus more closely on your fat and total food intake to get back on track.

> "I am always aware of what I am eating. I keep a mental track of what I have consumed."
>
> —Anne Y.

The Three Fs to Avoid

The thin people surveyed reported that they avoid the three Fs: fast, fried, and fake foods. They all ate these foods occasionally but not as a regular staple in their diets. They cited reasons such as wanting to set a good example for their children and not feeling well after eating these types of foods. All thin people surveyed complained that these foods were too high in fat content.

Thin people avoid fast food restaurants because of the limited number of healthy options available. Most thin people surveyed reported that they only occasionally dined at fast food restaurants and considered it to be a "treat." When they did eat fast food, they would sometimes choose a low-fat choice such as a grilled chicken sandwich, without the mayo, plus French fries. On other occasions, they might choose one higher fat item, such as a double cheeseburger, but skip the side orders. Many fried foods add unnecessary fat whereas the baked versions taste just as good. One thin person reported that she only ate fried foods at home where she could bake them. She said that her baked French fries are as good as any restaurants. Suggestions for making oven-fried favorites are included in Chapter 15.

Fake foods are all highly processed and refined foods. There are a variety of foods included in this category. Those that thin people tended to limit or altogether avoid were potato chips, prepackaged snack cakes, white bread, and sugar-laden beverages. These foods tend to add calories and fat, and very little nutritional value.

All carbohydrates are not created equal

When we talk about consuming carbohydrates, we need to first clarify a few terms. Carbohydrates can be complex or simple. Complex carbohydrates include all fruit, vegetables, legumes, beans, and whole grains. These grains include wheat, rye, oats or oatmeal, barley, and rice. Some complex carbohydrates are refined. In the refining process, the bran and germ have been removed from whole grains. Refined carbohydrates include white flour, everything made using white flour (such as white bread, cake, and bakery products), and white rice. Simple carbohydrates include sugar, honey, candy, regular soda, and other items made using sugar or syrups.

Calories derived from simple carbohydrates are often called "empty calories" because these foods lack essential amino acids, vitamins, and minerals. You will discover that some sugary candy is fat free, such as licorice ropes and gummy bears. Be aware that these treats still contain a substantial number of calories and should be limited. A good rule to follow is to limit your intake of calories from candy and other sweets to less than 200 total calories per day.

Complex carbohydrates are the preferred energy source over refined and simple carbohydrates. Complex carbohydrates contribute fiber and many essential nutrients, whereas refined grains have been stripped of most of their healthy qualities. The fiber found in the whole grains will also help lower elevated LDL cholesterol levels.

Simple carbohydrates contribute extra calories but little nutritional value. The sugar found in complex carbohydrates takes longer to leave the bloodstream, and therefore minimizes the drastic drop in blood sugars that occur shortly after the consumption of simple carbohydrates.

When you search for bread or cereals that are a good source of complex carbohydrates and fiber, the word *whole* should be the first word listed on the ingredient list. It may say whole wheat or whole oats on the front of the package, but make sure to check the ingredient list as well. Brownberry breads and Natural Ovens are both companies that use whole grains in their excellent tasting bread products.

Some cereals that are made using whole grain ingredients include Cheerios, Quaker Oat Squares, Bran Flakes, Raisin Bran, Wheaties, Total, Shredded Wheat, Frosted Shredded Wheat, Grape Nuts, and Grape Nut Flakes. Most hot cereals are good, whole grain choices, such as oatmeal, instant oatmeal, Cream of Wheat, Malt O' Meal, and wheat Farina. Good choices for crackers include 100 percent stone ground whole wheat crackers, Wasa crispbreads, Triscuits, and reduced fat Triscuits.

Sugar/Fat Combination

The sugar/fat combination is the best food combination for fat storage. When you eat or drink something that has a lot of sugar, it raises your blood sugar level, which causes an insulin surge. This release of insulin into the bloodstream is similar to a "lock and key" effect, opening up the door to the fat cells. When you consume fat following or in combination with the sugar, the fat is then more easily stored in your fat cells.

All high-protein and sugar-busting diets are based on this premise. The key is that if you consume something high in sugar, do not follow it with something that is also high in fat. The high-protein plans say that if you don't eat sugary foods at all, then you can eat the fat.

Your main goal is to keep the sugar separate from the fat. If you are eating a pepperoni and cheese pizza, avoid drinking a regular soda or lemonade with it. Drink water with your meal and then drink your soda two hours later if you still desire it. (The soda becomes more of a dessert.) Of course pizza and soda aren't recommended for optimal health, but if you are going to consume both on occasion, keep them apart.

Donuts are one of the best foods for fat storage. A donut recipe combines sugar and fat, with the added bonus of being deep-fried in grease. One donut can have as many as 40 grams of fat. Before choosing a donut, imagine it going into your mouth and moving directly to your hips.

Chapter 8:
Summary of Steps to Follow to Become a Thin Person

1. Limit your intake of fat to 30 to 40 grams per day for a woman and to 40 to 50 grams per day for a man.
2. Figure out how many fat grams are in your favorite foods.
3. Limit the three Fs: fast, fried, and fake.
4. Avoid the sugar/fat combination.
5. Choose complex carbohydrates over simple.
6. Remember: It's all about choices!

CHAPTER 9

Thin People Don't Go to a Restaurant or Party Starving

Your mother always said that snacking before a meal would "spoil your appetite." Spoiling your appetite slightly is desirable before going to a restaurant or party.

Stay in Control of Your Eating

Have you ever noticed that when you go to a restaurant feeling very hungry, you usually end up leaving the restaurant feeling stuffed? The reason is that when hungry, you are more likely to order an appetizer, eat from the breadbasket, order a higher-fat entree, and then eat dessert too.

You might notice that you feel a little out of control with respect to what, how much, and how fast you eat. By the time you get to the dessert cart, you think, "Oh what the heck, I've already blown it. I might as well have dessert too!" You are already planning to start a new diet tomorrow. This is a classic example of the overweight person's all-or-nothing mentality.

The thin person will focus on the conversation and the people she is dining with, while slowly enjoying and really tasting her food. How does she manage to stay so in control? Let's discuss the strategies that she uses.

Eat Before You Dine

If you find that you arrive at a restaurant very hungry, order a low-fat appetizer such as a tomato- or broth-based soup or tomato juice. This will help take the edge off of your appetite and put you back in control of your food choices and eating speed.

Ideally, you should eat a small snack an hour or two before going to the restaurant so that you will feel slightly hungry, yet still in control. A snack that consists mostly of complex carbohydrates, such as a banana or a slice of whole grain toast, is ideal. A more substantial snack that includes protein and fat will take longer to digest and may result in your not being hungry at all, which is not desirable.

Low-fat Menu Choices

When you are in control of your appetite, you will find that it is much easier to make healthy choices. The leanest cuts of red meat include those with the word choice or loin, such as tenderloin. Chicken without the skin, fish, and seafood are usually good low-fat choices. Some fish are higher in fat, such as salmon or trout, but are also high in omega-3 fatty acids, which are heart-healthy fats.

Choose your entrees dry broiled (no butter), baked, poached, steamed, or barbequed. Avoid foods that are breaded and fried. Often this cooking method is implied when you see the descriptive terms "crispy" or "golden brown" listed on the menu. Studies have shown that men tend to consume the majority of fat and calories in their diets from fatty meats and fried foods.

Salads are great starters, provided you practice the dipping technique with the salad dressing. Vegetables, including baked potatoes, are often good choices as long as butter has not been added. Adding your own toppings to your food will also help you stay in control of the fat and calories.

Don't be afraid to ask for your food to be prepared without added fats or dressings on the side. This is a request that is made often by those who frequent restaurants, especially the thin people we all should mimic. The more you practice making such special requests, the quicker these words will become a regular part of your vocabulary.

Portion Sizes

Keep in mind that a supper meal at a restaurant is typically double the portion size of the lunch meal. Does this mean Americans need more food and calories later in the evening? No, you actually need fewer calories in the evening since your body is gradually slowing its metabolism. Most European cultures eat their largest meal at noon, which allows most of their daily calories to be burned before the end of the day.

To control portion size in a restaurant, try one of the following techniques: Divide your meal in half, only eating the portion on one side of your plate and ask for a to-go box for the rest. If you don't feel disciplined enough to do this, ask that half of your meal be boxed to-go before your meal is even served. Another alternative is to split an entree with a friend to cut the portion size in half.

You're Satisfied. What Should You Do?

While you slowly eat your meal, pay attention to your appetite. When you notice that you are no longer hungry, put your fork down. Request that the remaining food be wrapped up to take home. If you don't want to take the leftover food home, cover your plate with your napkin. The waiter will know you've finished your meal and will clear your plate from the table. This will prevent you from continuing to pick at your food even though you are no longer hungry.

Low-fat Desserts May Be Hazardous to Your Health

Beware of low-fat desserts. Sweet items that are advertised as low-fat are generally very high in calories. Removing the fat from a dessert usually takes out much of the flavor. To make the dessert taste good again, extra syrup and sugar are added. The result is that the calories weigh in almost as high as the original dessert. You are much better off having a taste or two of a regular, more satisfying dessert (remember Jackie O?).

Most restaurants have a small cup of sherbet or fresh fruit available even if it is not listed on the menu. Fruit satisfies your craving for something sweet because it contains fructose, or "fruit sugar," and your body's cells do not know the difference. Alternately, a piece of hard candy or a stick of gum is sometimes all you need to feel satisfied or get that garlic taste out of your mouth. Keep gum available for such occasions.

How to Handle Buffet-Style Restaurants

When going to a buffet-style restaurant, people tend to eat far more than they need. This type of restaurant can be a disaster zone for members of the clean plate club. You will have plenty of opportunity to practice leaving food on your plate. Your main goal when eating from a buffet is to focus on sampling the foods, nibbling like a mouse rather than feasting like a king.

You need to control food portions for yourself at a buffet, and it will be much easier if you are not starving when you get there. Make sure to eat a snack an hour or two before you arrive.

Don't be fooled into thinking that by only eating from the salad bar you are making healthy choices. You can easily build a salad with enough food for a family of five! Others make several return trips, topping the salad scales with thousands of calories and loads of fat. Remember, there are just as many fat grams lurking at the salad bar as there are at the other stations of the buffet.

In fact, you may benefit from skipping the salad bar altogether to avoid eating to the point of uncomfortable, which is your number one goal when attending a buffet meal. You should then eat more fruits and vegetables at your next meal or snack.

Give yourself permission to try anything that you want from any of the buffet tables. If you really want the fried chicken, mashed potatoes, and ice cream, have them. Take the skin off of the chicken and use a small amount of gravy instead of butter plus gravy to make your selection a little less calorie-laden. The key here is to really enjoy the food, eating it slowly with control. Don't inhale it so that you can hurry back for more. Think of yourself as a food connoisseur. Food-tasters rarely eat a whole anything!

Evaluating Your Success

Make a note as to how long it takes for you to get hungry again after eating at an unlimited buffet. It may take an hour or so longer than usual, depending on how much fat was in the foods that you chose. Fat remains in the stomach longer than carbohydrates. If you start to notice hunger signals just a few hours after eating, you may not have eaten enough volume or protein. Your goal should be to start feeling hungry again approximately three to four hours after completing the meal.

One thin person commented that when dining at a buffet-style restaurant, she only goes up to the food tables once. She takes exactly what she wants to eat the first time and never lets any of her foods touch. This strategy prevents her from overfilling her plate and helps with portion control.

The first time you eat at a buffet in this manner, you will leave the restaurant feeling a little strange. You may question whether you got your money's worth. You will find yourself smiling when all of your companions are complaining about feeling stuffed and uncomfortable. You may feel slightly guilty when you are hungry a few hours later, but don't. Take it as a clue that your body digested the food and is ready for more. Learn to deal with these new feelings. Being classified as a thin person is well worth it.

Some people find that it is difficult to dine out when they are first learning new, thin-friendly eating habits. Others will say it is much easier to eat at a restaurant than at home because eating in public keeps them more accountable. However you initially feel, keep in mind that you live in the real world and eventually need to learn how to eat like a thin person in all environments.

How Thin People Eat at Parties

Thin people approach parties the same way that they approach restaurant dining. They arrive at the party slightly hungry, yet are in control of their appetite and food choices. Most thin people avoid socializing around the food tables at a party. Standing near the food only entices you to consume extra servings. Most thin people fill a plate of food and then move away from the food area to eat it.

When observing thin people at a party, you will notice that they really taste the food. They savor it in their mouth, chew it well and pause before taking another bite. They appear to be very sophisticated and in control, but the truth is that they are not overly hungry.

Alcohol May Hinder Weight Loss

Consuming alcohol is counterproductive to weight loss for several reasons. First, at 7 calories per gram, alcohol is much closer in calories to fat (9 calories per gram) than protein or carbohydrates (4 calories per gram). The calories add up quickly in these beverages.

Second, alcohol has been found to slow your metabolism. Just one beverage will decrease your metabolism by up to 36 percent at the next meal. Alcohol also increases fat storage because of the surge of insulin in the bloodstream following ingestion.

Alcohol, especially on an empty stomach, will actually increase your appetite as your blood sugars start to fall (in reaction to the insulin surge) shortly after the beverage has been consumed. This usually leads to an increase in the amount of food and number of calories you consume.

If you eat a snack an hour or so before attending the party, your stomach will not be completely empty and alcohol will not affect you as abruptly. Having more than a few drinks, however, may again lead to excess eating (to say nothing of the several hundred extra calories from the cocktails alone).

Finally, a "what the heck" attitude may set in as your inhibitions are lessened with the relaxing effects of the alcohol, which is categorized as a depressant. Bottom line: Drink alcohol in moderation, if at all. Moderation is typically recognized as one drink per day for a woman and no more than two drinks per day for a man.

Food Choices at the Party

Hosts for parties are more concerned with the palatability of the food, than its fat content. For this reason, consider eating a light meal or a full snack before attending the party to increase your ability to resist the high-fat menu items.

Fresh fruit and vegetables are always healthy choices for weight control at a party; just beware of the accompanying dip that will surely be loaded with fat and calories. Pretzels are low in fat but contain a lot of sodium, which could cause the dial on your scale to be up the next morning. If you eat salty items, plan to drink extra water to help flush the excess sodium out of your body.

Be a minimalist when it comes to the fried foods being served as well as those stuffed with cream cheese fillings or covered with cheese. You do not need to deprive yourself of these tasty foods, just keep your portion sizes small. These types of foods are perfect for you to continue the art of eating like a food connoisseur.

Another option to ensure low-fat choices at the party is to bring one. By making low-fat substitutions to your recipe (see Chapter 15), you can be sure that there will be at least one healthy food available. If you choose the right substitutions and additions, nobody will even know that your dish is low fat.

Chapter 9:
Summary of Steps to Follow to Become a Thin Person

1. Eat a snack or light meal before going to a restaurant or party.

2. Make low-fat choices.

3. Request that all sauces and salad dressings be served on the side and use the dipping technique.

4. Eat slowly with control, focusing on the conversation.

5. Stop eating when you are no longer hungry.

6. Ask for a "to-go" box for the leftovers.

7. At buffets, stop eating when you are no longer hungry.

CHAPTER 10

Thin People
Eat Chocolate

*Chocolate, oh so decadent and enticing
...what a lovely treat.*

The All-Or-Nothing Way of Thinking

Overweight people tend to have the all-or-nothing mentality. They will either not touch the brownies or will eat most of the pan, promising themselves that this will be the last time they ever eat chocolate. The thin person will typically have one brownie and savor every bite, knowing that she is only going to eat one.

The thin person avoids depriving herself of the foods she loves. The exception is if brownies happen to be a "trigger food" (see page 68). Deprivation is a form of punishment, whereas eating should be an enjoyable experience.

Letting go of the all-or-nothing mentality takes practice. Allow yourself to eat one piece of chocolate and then remove the temptation, or take yourself away from the area where the chocolates are located. (It doesn't have to be chocolate, but any food that is a treat for you.)

When you put a treat into your mouth, practice the art of sensual eating by really savoring it. Tell yourself that you can have another piece but not today. Eventually, you will be satisfied with just one piece of chocolate, and you can experience it every day if you like. You are now enjoying sinful treats in the manner that a thin person would.

Thin People Know Their Trigger Foods

Thin people know which foods are their "out-of-control" or "trigger" foods. These are the foods that a person feels she cannot stop eating once she starts or it triggers an eating binge. This food can be anything from chips with dip to homemade chocolate chip cookies. The specific food is usually different for each individual.

Change your way of thinking about your trigger food. Instead of thinking that you cannot stop eating it once you start, think that you are the one who chooses to continue to eat the food. In the second scenario, you are in control, not the food. Remember, you are ultimately responsible for what goes into your mouth and body.

> "I don't buy the foods that I consider to be my 'out-of-control' foods. I only have them when I am out for dinner or on special occasions."
> —Jill R.

Portion Sizes

When controlling your portion size, you must avoid eating any food directly out of the bag or container. This is especially true while enjoying your favorite foods, but imperative for your personal trigger foods.

Keep in mind that your stomach is only as large as your fist. This means that the amount of food that you put into your body at one time does not need to exceed this volume. Place all of the food that you plan to eat on your plate before you start eating, and put the serving containers of food away. This will help you realize the volume that you are eating.

It takes your stomach 20 minutes to signal to your brain that it is satisfied. If you eat your meal too fast, you may still feel hun-

gry even though your portion of food is gone. Wait out the re-
mainder of the 20 minutes for your hunger to subside. Don't think
that you need to eat more food.

Carbohydrate-Sensitive Individuals

Some people are more sensitive to the effects of carbohydrates,
in particular, the simple and refined carbohydrates. They find that
the more simple or refined carbohydrates they eat the more of
these types of carbohydrates they crave. These people are sometimes called "carbohydrate sensitive" or "carbohydrate addicts."

A diet that is high in simple carbohydrates and processed foods
will often produce rebound, low blood sugars. Low blood sugars
cause intense cravings for even more of these processed foods,
such as white bread, potato chips, snack cakes, soda, and other
sweets. When you eat too many refined carbohydrates, your blood
sugar quickly rises. This causes the pancreas to secrete extra insulin into the bloodstream. The blood sugar levels then drop,
increasing the urge to eat even more of the sweets and processed
foods.

To break this cycle, which often leads to excessive weight gain,
you must decrease your intake of simple carbohydrates and refined foods. The fewer of these items you eat, the less intense your
cravings will be. You will experience fewer fluctuations in blood
sugars, which will help you feel more in control of your food
choices.

Chapter 10:
Summary of Steps to Follow to Become a Thin Person

1. Eat your favorite, high-fat food, in small portions.

2. Really savor your favorite food in your mouth.

3. Do not deprive yourself. Remember moderation.

4. Avoid or limit your personal trigger foods.

5. Limit your intake of simple sugars and carbohydrates if you consider yourself to be carbohydrate sensitive.

CHAPTER 11

Thin People Drink Water

Water is essential for life and weight loss.

Why Do I Need to Drink Water?

You were probably instructed to drink a lot of water while following diets in the past. You may have consumed the water without knowing why it was important. Water is your secret weapon against fat. You cannot mobilize your fat stores without water. It is needed in the basic biochemical equation for fat metabolism. Both water and oxygen are needed to break stored fat down into the smaller molecules the body uses for energy.

> "The secret to staying thin is water, water, and more water."
>
> —Stephanie F.

How Much Water Do I Need to Drink?

Start by drinking 8 cups, or 64 ounces, of water each day. For every 25 pounds of excess weight above your ideal body weight, drink an additional cup of water. If you have 50 pounds to lose, drink 10 cups (80 ounces) of water each day.

Observe your urine to evaluate if you are drinking enough water. Ideally, your urine should be very pale in color. It should be clear, not cloudy, and without odor. Be aware that multivitamins will intensify the color of your urine, as will some fortified cereals, such as Total.

Sixty-four ounces may sound like a lot of water if you are not currently a big water drinker. Once you become accustomed to drinking this volume, you will find that it does get easier. Your body will even start to crave additional water. Those who drink inadequate amounts of water are rarely thirsty. You will find that the more water you drink, the thirstier you will be.

Your body's need for water increases in hot and dry weather, as well as with physical activity. In these situations, it is a good idea to drink some water every 15 to 30 minutes even if you do not feel thirsty. A healthy adult can survive weeks without food but just a few days without water.

Water Retention

For a healthy person who does not have any heart problems or kidney failure, water retention should not be a normal occurrence. If you have a problem with water retention, you will notice that this condition lessens or goes away altogether once your intake of water is up to the body's desired level. Your body retains fluids because it perceives that there is a shortage of water due to inadequate intake. Your body is attempting to hang on to as much of the water as possible to survive.

Your body will go through a period of adjustment as you begin to supply it with the extra water that it needs. Once your body is satisfied that the water shortage is over, it will release the fluid that is has been storing in your extremities. You will feel lighter and less water-logged in a few days. You will also drop several pounds. If you have retained water in the past, you may come to believe water is the miracle that you've been seeking because it is common to reach a newfound energy level.

Drink your first cup or two of water first thing in the morning. This helps flush any retained fluids from the previous day and helps increase your thirst for water all day long. Most people find that it is easiest to drink this first glass quickly, even if they are not thirsty, before doing anything else to start their day.

What if I don't like water?

Not everyone will enjoy drinking water. Here are a few tips that may make your new water habit less uncomfortable. Use a straw to help you drink quickly. This is especially helpful if you are having a difficult time consuming the required amount in a day. Most large sports bottles hold 4 cups of water. You only have to drink two full bottles to reach your minimum goal of 8 cups of water per day.

You may find it helpful to fill a pitcher with 8 cups of water and put it into the refrigerator before going to bed at night. The pitcher should be empty by the end of the next day. If it is not empty, refill it and start over the next day. It will get easier as drinking water becomes a habit.

Experiment with different water temperatures to determine what you like best. Some research concludes that consuming cold water is best. You will burn more calories because your body attempts to warm it to body temperature. This increase in burned calories is minimal, so don't drink ice-cold water if you prefer tepid. The most important thing is to drink it.

To make your water more enjoyable, try adding lemon or lime wedges or a slice of cucumber. You can also try adding a splash of fruit juice to give it a boost. Avoid substituting other beverages for water. You are fooling yourself if you believe that your skim milk, fruit juice, or diet soda count as water. Sure, you are getting some water from these beverages, but you may also be getting extra calories or caffeine too. Aim to drink your full 64-plus ounces of water from actual water and think of your additional fluid sources as a bonus.

Caffeine and Alcohol

Beverages that contain caffeine have a diuretic effect on the body, causing the body to excrete more water than it should, which could potentially leave you dehydrated. Not only should you not count caffeinated beverages toward your water intake, but you should also consume more water to compensate for the extra fluids that are pulled from your body. For each cup of coffee you drink, plan to drink an additional cup of water.

Drinking decaffeinated coffee or tea is not the solution. They still contain a small amount of caffeine, as well as tannins. Tannins also act as diuretics to a lesser degree. For every cup of decaffeinated coffee, tea, or caffeinated soda you drink, consume approximately ½ cup of additional water.

Another type of beverage that has a similar but intensified diuretic effect on the body is alcohol. Dehydration is the main reason that people experience a hangover after a night of consuming alcoholic beverages. To prevent this loss of excess body fluids, which causes the headache, alternate each alcoholic beverage with a glass of water.

Additional Benefits of Drinking Water

Now you know the most important reason to drink your water every day. You cannot lose body fat without supplying enough water to your body. There are several other reasons why you need to drink enough water:

- Water helps you rid your body of metabolized fat and other waste materials. The only way to remove the stored fat and toxins from your body is through urine or sweat. If you are sweating a lot, you again need more water to replace what you have lost.

- Water keeps the skin healthy and resilient. You must replace water frequently because you lose about 2½ quarts a day.

Drinking enough water helps minimize sagging skin as you lose weight.

- Muscle contains a large percentage of water. Drinking water helps maintain proper muscle tone.

- Sufficient water intake will help relieve and prevent constipation. Stools will pass more frequently and without strain if the proper amount of fluid is being consumed. Fiber alone will not cure constipation.

- Water helps suppress the appetite. Many people eat in relation to thirst instead of actual hunger.

- Water is essential for digestion, absorption of vitamins and minerals, circulation, excretion, transporting nutrients, building tissue, and maintaining body temperature.

Older individuals may say that they are never thirsty. This is because as you get older, your thirst mechanism becomes faulty. You need to drink the water even though your body may not be sending the signal to drink. By the time most people become thirsty, they are already slightly dehydrated.

You will find that when you increase your water consumption, your energy level drastically increases. This is especially true if you are currently walking around in a semi-dehydrated state. You may naturally decrease your intake of caffeinated beverages as you increase your intake of water. This helps eliminate the energy surges and drains that you may experience in response to caffeine.

Be aware that you will need to frequent the restroom much more often as you increase your water intake. Most people only seem to find this an obstacle in the beginning. It could be that they just get used to going more often. If you are concerned about waking up in the middle of the night to go to the bathroom, try to finish drinking all of your water prior to 6:00 P.M.

Chapter 11:
Summary of Steps to Follow to Become a Thin Person

1. Drink a minimum of 8 cups of water every day.

2. Check to make sure that your urine is a clear, pale color without odor.

3. If you choose to drink caffeine or alcohol, make sure you drink extra water to compensate for the diuretic effect of these beverages.

CHAPTER 12

Thin People Move Their Bodies

You do not need to love moving your body...
Just enjoy it more than carrying excess body fat.

Remembering How to Enjoy Movement

In Chapter 2, we discussed starting your metabolism by eating breakfast. The second most important method of increasing your metabolic rate is with movement (exercise). Exercise is the single best predictor of long-term success with permanent weight loss. By increasing your heart rate and breathing while using major muscle groups, you increase the rate at which your body burns calories. The real calorie burn continues for 8-24 hours after you finish your exercise (after-burn).

Most people are turned off by the word "exercise" because it sounds like hard work. It doesn't have to be. Do you remember what you liked to do as a child? Did you enjoy biking or swimming or doing the hula-hoop? Choose an activity that you enjoyed as a child and try it again as an adult. You will be surprised to find that you may still love this activity. Connie G. found that when she began riding a bicycle as an adult, she felt like a kid again.

Think of your exercise as movement or "playing" instead of exercising. All three terms are used throughout this book. Choose the term you are the most comfortable with when referring to your own body movement.

One thin woman called her exercise sessions her "mama time" because she was taking time for herself. She learned that it was acceptable for her to take some time away from her children without any guilt. This is called "healthy selfishness," and it is beneficial to the whole family.

"Healthy selfishness" is when you do something for yourself that takes you temporarily away from others who depend on you. You need to realize that if you don't take care of yourself first, you will not be able to physically or mentally take care of others. Remember the flight attendant on the airplane telling you that, in the event of an emergency, you should always put your own oxygen mask on before helping your children? This is an example of healthy selfishness. It is acceptable for you to take time for yourself to exercise on a regular basis. You will be an even better care giver once you return.

When to Move Your Body

Morning is the best time for most people to exercise because of their busy schedules. Too many excuses and unplanned events surface later in the day. Your children may have sports or school programs that you need to attend. You have bills to pay, laundry to do, and a kitchen to clean. Plus a friend may call or stop over to talk. Television shows are also much more interesting in the evening than at 6 A.M. Fitness club trainers will tell you that those who exercise in the morning are 90 to 100 percent consistent in their exercise schedules, while those who exercise later in the day are much less regimented.

> "I like to exercise every day. I try to do it first thing in the morning, if not then, as soon as I get home from work."
>
> —Deb F.

By exercising in the morning, you only have to take one shower and get ready for the day once. Morning exercisers can roll right out of bed and be ready to exercise in approximately 2 minutes. If you choose to take the time to brush your teeth and comb your hair it might take a few minutes more. But trust me, no one expects you to be looking your best at 6:00 in the morning!

Organize and lay out your clothes and shoes the night before to simplify your morning routine. If you have to dig in the closet for 10 minutes to find your walking shoes in the morning, you will become frustrated and waste precious time. Place your clothes and shoes in the bathroom. When your alarm goes off in the morning, get out of bed and head for the bathroom. You can be fully dressed by the time you stand up from using the facilities.

Never push the snooze button on your alarm clock. It helps to position your alarm clock on the opposite side of the room so that you need to actually get out of your bed to shut it off. Then, don't look back at your bed. Go directly to the bathroom. Looking back seems to magically pull you back into your bed. Also avoid talking to yourself. You will find yourself making promises to exercise later, which never seems to happen.

After you are done with your 30 minutes of activity, you will be very proud of yourself. You will find that you have more energy all morning long, much more energy than if you had slept your precious exercise time away. Your body will also be burning more calories throughout the day.

Exercising later in the day means that you have to tote clothes, hair supplies, and makeup with you to work. If you find the time to exercise in the evening, you will probably need to shower before going to bed, which works fine for some people and does free up the shower for others in the morning.

If you already have an established exercise routine that starts later in the day, that is great and you do not need to change it. Keep up the good work! Consistency, regardless of the time of the day, is the key.

Frequency and Duration of Movement

The ideal goal is to move your body for at least 30 minutes most days of the week. To meet weight-loss goals faster, the goal should be increased to 45 to 60 minutes most days of the week. Most research agrees that after 60 minutes, not much additional benefit is added and you substantially increase your risk of injury.

Walking 30 minutes every day will burn approximately 250 calories per day (based on a person who weighs 155 pounds and walks briskly), which translates to a calorie deficit of 3,500 calories every two weeks or a weight loss of 1 pound every two weeks without any changes to your diet. You could lose 26 pounds in one year by just adding 30 minutes of exercise to your day. If you chose to walk for an hour each day of the week, you would burn enough calories to lose one pound per week or 52 pounds in a year—again, without any dietary changes.

> "My diet isn't perfect, but I always exercise at least four to five times per week."
> —Debbie R.

Wearing a pedometer can be a good gauge of your daily movement. Just be aware that some pedometers, usually those in the $3 to $10 range will count steps with even the slightest of movement, indicating that you're being more active than you truly are. Since weight loss is your goal, you should aim to take approximately 10,000 steps every day. This translates to walking 4½ miles.

The majority of the thin people interviewed said they felt something was "missing" from their day if they didn't exercise. All of the thin people, without exception, described themselves as active people. Wasting energy, by keeping busy or active, burns extra calories all day long and helps to keep your metabolism burning at its maximum.

To burn extra calories, stand instead of sitting while talking on the telephone. Do leg lifts while brushing your teeth for some extra toning. Don't wait until you have 10 items to take downstairs, take each item down as it appears. Every single thing you do to waste calories will help add to the calorie deficit that you are hoping to grow.

Schedule your activity into your day as if it were an appointment. Put it in your date book or on your calendar along with your other commitments. Schedule it at a time when you will realistically do it. Scheduling will help you think of your exercise time as non-negotiable. It will also prevent you from scheduling something else during your allotted exercise time.

Don't skip exercise more than two days in a row. The first day that you don't exercise you will think about it and wish that you had made the time to do it. You will think about the extra energy you had the day before and how good you felt. The second day you skip your exercise session, you will still think about the positive benefits without as much remorse. After skipping your third day of exercise, exercise will become "work" again in your mind. These three skipped sessions can quickly turn into weeks and months.

Don't think of your exercise time as time lost. Think of it as an investment in yourself. You are much more productive during the rest of your day after getting your blood pumping and supplying your brain with the extra oxygen that it needs for increased concentration.

If you plan to walk, jog, or bike, use your car to map out some different routes with varying distances. On the days when you are short of time, choose one of the shorter distances. Save the longer routes for the days when you have ample time and

> "I do consider myself to be an active person, chasing after my two- and four-year-old children all day, although I only officially exercise two times each week. If I am feeling sluggish, I will walk on the treadmill, which perks me up."
>
> —Jennie K.

energy. How long it takes you to complete each route will also be a good gauge for you to measure your progress.

When your exercise begins to seem too easy, the health benefits decrease. Adjust your routine to increase the amount of time you spend doing your exercise or the distance that you cover. You need to work your body longer or at a higher intensity to elevate your heart rate and get the same metabolism-boosting effects as you previously did. This is the only down side of becoming physically fit. That and having to buy new clothes!

Set Goals

By setting goals, you will keep yourself motivated and constantly working toward something. Your goals may change weekly, such as exercising three times per week for the next four weeks. An excellent method of tracking a goal like this is to hang a calendar in your bathroom or any other location where you will see it several times each day. When you finish your activity, place a sticker on the day or draw a big star with a marker.

At a glance, you will be constantly reminded of how many exercise sessions you have completed each week and month. When the month is over, tally your stickers or stars, write the total on the bottom of the page (such as 19 out of 30), and flip the calendar page to the next month. You start fresh with each new month, but you can look back at your progress anytime.

You will probably start to notice that the stress in your life decreases as the number of stars on your calendar increases. You are not imagining this. Exercise produces natural mood-lifters, called endorphins. They act much in the same

"I have never learned to love exercise. I do, however, love the energy and feeling of optimal health that I experience following each daily walk."

—Rhonda H.

way that anti-depressants do, only without the negative side effects of the drugs.

Some people may choose to set long-range goals, such as participating in an event. This could be a 5-kilometer walk or even a full marathon or triathlon. Set your goal according to your comfort level and what you wish to achieve. Again, you don't need to love your exercise. You only need to like it better than being overweight, constantly feeling sluggish, and dying prematurely. If you like exercise better than the alternative, get started. Start moving your body today!

Thin People Lift Weights

Your aging body does not retain its muscle mass without some form of weight bearing exercise. Your metabolism naturally begins to decrease with age, mostly due to a loss of lean muscle mass, at a rate of approximately 20 percent per decade. This means that if you were burning approximately 2,000 calories per day when you were in your twenties, in your thirties you can expect to burn 1,900 calories per day and only 1,800 in your forties.

You will continue to burn approximately 100 calories less per day as each decade passes. This metamorphosis tends to begin for most people in their early to mid-thirties. The good news is that this decrease in metabolism can be avoided. By lifting weights, you can retain and even build new lean muscle mass.

When you begin lifting weights, you may notice that your weight goes up slightly. This weight gain is only temporary. As you increase your metabolism because of the increase in your lean muscle mass, your body will begin burning more calories all day long. This will help promote fat loss, which will in turn bring the scale back down below your starting weight.

One thin person stated that lifting weights was like the "fountain of youth" for her. She explained that her 45-year-old body had been transformed since she started adding weight lifting to her exercise routine. She felt sculpted. Her current routine includes walking 30 minutes daily and lifting weights three times a week for approximately 30 to 45 minutes. You can hire a personal trainer to help you set up a weight-lifting routine that is right for you without a huge financial commitment.

You do not need to become a professional body builder to appreciate the benefits of lifting weights. Lifting weights two to three times per week is all that is required to prevent the muscle loss that occurs naturally with age. You can do your weight lifting at home with a few inexpensive hand weights and a good fitness (toning) video.

Begin to "Waste" Energy

Learn to burn extra calories all day long by making small changes in your current lifestyle. Something as simple as doing leg lifts while you brush your teeth can help you tone your muscles, burn a few calories, and raise your metabolism. Taking the stairs as a rule instead of ever using the elevators or escalators is also a great calorie waster.

A recent research study found that when participants avoided going through all drive-throughs, including fast food restaurants, the bank, and dry cleaners, they lost an average of 12 pounds in just one year. They were still allowed to go in if they wanted to visit these places, but they needed to get out of their car. What a simple lifestyle change!

One of the easiest ways to increase your calorie expenditure is to park your car farther away from your destination. If you always choose the parking spot that is the farthest away from work or the store, you will burn hundreds of extra calories each day. Some people will park a full six blocks away from work, which will add an extra mile of walking every day.

Lunch breaks usually allow enough time to catch a quick 10-minute walk around the parking lot or block. The fresh air, in addition to the feel-good hormones (endorphins) that are released by your body, will give you an extra boost of energy as you approach the afternoon hours.

> "I always take the stairs instead of the elevator."
>
> —Liza M.

Isometric exercises are when you contract a specific muscle or group of muscles and hold them in the contracted state for a period of time. This could include squeezing your buttocks or gluteal muscles while standing in line at the store. Or holding your stomach muscles tight (pushing your lower back into the back of your seat) every time you are waiting at a red light while in your car. These isometric exercises can be performed anywhere, usually quite inconspicuously to those around you.

The more you waste energy in the form of calories, the faster you will meet your weight-loss goals. Just as a few handfuls of chips or candy here and there add up calories quickly, the few extra calories you burn with these energy wasters quickly accumulate too. Think about how fast your goals will be reached if you cut out those extra calories and burn a few more!

Thin People Get Extra Oxygen

As mentioned previously, the breakdown of body fat requires two components, water and oxygen. You need to drink water to facilitate this breakdown. Now, what about the oxygen?

Oxygen is required to break a fat cell down into parts small enough for the body to use as an energy source. How do you get this needed oxygen? By breathing, of course. But, you need more oxygen than you take in through normal, everyday breathing. Two methods to acquire the additional oxygen you need are: (1) aerobic exercise and (2) deep breathing.

Aerobic Exercise

The word aerobic means "with oxygen." You need to perform exercise during which the body consumes extra oxygen. This includes any activity that elevates your heart rate and increases your rate of breathing. It can be walking, biking, jumping rope, doing fitness videos, or any other aerobic activity that you choose.

This exercise is the playtime or movement of your body that we were discussing previously in this chapter, not additional exercise. The recommended 30 minutes of movement most days of the week provides the additional oxygen you need to break down stored body fat.

Deep Breathing

The second method of acquiring the additional, needed oxygen is deep breathing. It is simple to do and can be done almost anywhere. All you need to do is focus on your breaths and breathe deeply for several minutes. Perform this task twice each day for a period of five minutes each time. If you can only do it for a couple of minutes, do it. It is much better than not doing it at all.

> "I feel that exercise is the most important habit I have that keeps me thin. Not because of the calories burned, but because I know that if my mind is healthy, I am able to keep my body healthy. It is all part of the big picture."
>
> —Anne F.

There are different deep breathing techniques that you can learn, but do not make this simple activity more complicated than it needs to be. Make sure you are using your stomach muscles during this exercise. Your stomach should expand (inflate) as you inhale and it should go in (deflate) as you exhale. Using your stomach muscles as you practice your deep breathing helps tighten them, which you will be able to see more clearly once you begin losing your excess abdominal fat.

Deep breathing also helps keep you alert because the extra oxygen goes to your brain. This is particularly helpful during a sluggish point in your day.

Deep breathing is a useful relaxation technique and can be considered a form of meditation (discussed in Chapter 13). Many people use deep breathing and meditation to help deal with the stress in their lives. You can do your breathing exercises anywhere. Just find a quiet area, close your eyes, and start breathing. Try to avoid letting negative thoughts pop into your head during this time.

One example of a simple breathing technique is called "square breathing." To square breath, you need to take a deep breath in for a count of five. You then hold this breath for a count of five. Next, slowly exhale for a count of five. Finally, hold the breath out for a count of five. Repeat this exercise 5 to 10 times, or until you begin to feel relaxed.

You may prefer to do your deep breathing exercises while lying down with your eyes closed. Playing quiet music can help create a peaceful setting for this activity as well. With these serene changes, the breathing exercise becomes a form of meditation, which can help lower your blood pressure and improve your mood. So start breathing deeply today and enjoy all of the wonderful benefits.

Chapter 12:
Summary of Steps to Follow to Become a Thin Person

1. Set your alarm to wake up 45 minutes earlier than usual.
2. Move your body for 30 minutes most mornings.
3. Lift weights two or three days per week to retain muscle mass.
4. Breathe deeply as you move your body.
5. Breathe deeply for five minutes twice each day.

CHAPTER 13

Thin People Rest Their Bodies

Sleep is essential to reach and maintain a healthy weight.

Importance of Sleep to Weight Loss

When trying to lose weight, research shows that sleep is as important as exercise and eating well. Research studies have revealed that those who do not get enough sleep tend to have more body fat. Part of the reason for this is because a lack of sleep can actually increase your appetite. Typically when you have an increased appetite as a result of inadequate sleep, you are not hungry for fruit and vegetables. Your body craves more calorie-dense foods, such as fatty, fried and fast foods. These calorie heavy foods are an easy way to pack on the excess pounds.

To encourage sleep (for those with insomnia), try eating a small, high-carbohydrate snack approximately 45 minutes before going to bed. A few crackers or a cup or two of popcorn is sufficient. The carbohydrates will increase your brain's production of serotonin, a neurotransmitter that causes a calming or sleepy effect on your body. Remember that ideally we would not eat during the three hours prior to going to sleep, but with insomnia, the lack of sleep will be more detrimental to your weight-loss efforts than eating a small serving of carbohydrates is.

Avoid caffeine and alcohol to promote optimal sleep patterns. Caffeine, being a stimulant, can actually prevent you from feeling tired when you are. Limit caffeine after early afternoon to prevent this. Alcohol has been found to help individuals initially fall asleep, but then they experience several periods of interrupted sleep throughout the night.

Regular exercise also helps prevent insomnia. Exercising in the early afternoon is the optimal time of day for people who have insomnia. Avoid exercising in the evening because it may increase your alertness and keep you awake.

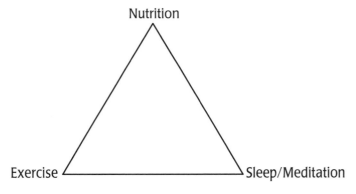

The Wellness Triangle

Nutrition

Exercise

Sleep/Meditation

The wellness triangle, shown above, represents the ultimate balance for good health in a person's life. When aspiring to become a thin person, each corner of the triangle needs to be in balance with the other two corners. If you pay attention to all three areas, you will achieve your health improvement goals.

Ideally, paying attention to the nutrition corner means that you are feeding your body healthy foods in small quantities throughout the day. This corner also includes a good intake of water, with limited caffeine and alcohol consumption. You are listening to your body and not over or under feeding it.

The exercise corner is in its ideal state when you are moving your body a minimum of 30 minutes most days of the week, while breathing deeply to take in extra oxygen. Lifting weights a few times each week also enhances the exercise corner. Burning more calories daily by being active is a bonus.

The sleep corner of the wellness triangle is optimal when you sleep an average of six and one-half to seven and one-half hours each night. This suggested amount of sleep time is backed up by recent research that revealed most individuals who slept for this length of time woke up feeling refreshed and alert. Sleeping more than eight hours per night was not recommended by this research.

Some individuals may find that they do not need this much sleep each night, whereas others will feel that they need more. Gauge how much sleep you personally need on how you feel upon waking. Keep a sleep journal for a week. Write down how much sleep you got each night versus how you felt the next morning.

This sleep, in a perfect world, is not restless, but sound and without interruptions. A lot of overweight people will find that they do not sleep in the perfect world. With excess weight, you may experience back aches or muscle cramps. Many individuals who are overweight will also experience sleep apnea. These problems will lessen with weight loss.

Meditation

Meditation is included in the sleep corner of the triangle, as it is a form of rest for both the mind and the body. Meditation helps quiet the mind so that it can focus, which will help your entire body experience a heightened sense of well-being. If you have a lot of stress in your life, you will find that meditation helps bring you back to your inner self by allowing you let go of the external details of your daily job and life.

We discussed square breathing in the last chapter, which is one form of meditation. Since you will be experiencing an increase in oxygen with either the deep, square breathing or other form of meditation, feel free to choose one or the other to perform each day. It is not necessary to do both.

Find a quiet place to meditate, where you can calm your mind and totally relax, as you strive to experience inner peace. Close your eyes. Breathe in through your nose slowly and then exhale slowly. A lot of people will find that repeating a chant word, such as "calm," over and over slowly, will help them feel more centered.

There are several excellent guided-imagery audiotapes or CDs that can help you relax and get into your meditative-state of well-being. See the suggested reading list at the end of Chapter 17 for suggestions.

Balance Your Triangle

If you neglect any one corner of the triangle, the triangle is out of balance and you are not in optimal health. For example, if you are not getting enough sleep to awake feeling refreshed and alert, you will have an increased appetite, causing you to eat more fast, processed, and refined foods. When you eat poorly, in addition to not having enough sleep, you will rarely have the energy to move your body or engage in exercise.

If you increase caffeine to compensate for the lack of sleep, the whole triangle is out of balance. Because of the caffeine, you will most likely not experience a good night's sleep the next night either. Consequently, the cycle of eating poorly and not exercising continues.

To break this vicious cycle, you must balance the three corners of your wellness triangle. To begin, exercise to make your body physically tired. This will help you get a good night's sleep. After a good night's sleep, you will be able to control your appetite and improve the whole triangle.

A near-perfect scenario is that you sleep peacefully for seven hours at night. You wake up refreshed and go for a morning walk for at least 30 minutes. You then eat a balanced diet full of lean protein, whole grains, fruit and vegetables, drink plenty of water, and limit both caffeinated and alcoholic beverages. You dedicate a total of 10 minutes to meditation or deep breathing, where you quiet your mind. At the end of the day, you go to bed feeling tired and get another 7 hours restful sleep, going on to repeat this cycle the next day.

Chapter 13:
Summary of Steps to Follow to Become a Thin Person

1. Get enough sleep each night to awake refreshed and alert.

2. Envision the wellness triangle in your life daily.

3. Make time to either meditate or do your deep breathing for a total of 10 minutes each day.

CHAPTER 14

A Typical Day in the Life of a Thin Person

Let's pick the brain of the (enviable) Thin Person

The Thin Person: Maggie

Let's give our hypothetical thin person a name for the sake of this discussion. We will call her Maggie. Maggie is a typical thin person. She follows the majority of the steps that most thin people follow on a regular basis to help her maintain her sleek figure.

Each night before going to bed, Maggie sets her alarm to wake up one hour before the rest of her family wakes up. She places her alarm clock on the counter in the bathroom to force herself out of bed in the morning. Maggie sets her "mama-time" clothes on the bathroom counter and her walking shoes on the floor. This saves precious time and prevents the frustration of hunting for items in the morning when she is not yet awake.

Maggie's Morning

Maggie's alarm rings at 6:00 A.M. Without thinking, she mechanically gets out of bed and heads to the bathroom. She quietly closes the door behind her, turns on the light, and turns off the alarm clock. She knows better than to even look back at her bed once she is out of it. For the mere sight of her comfortable, warm bed is far too inviting and it will seem to beckon her to rejoin it. Maggie sits down on the commode as she begins to put her clothes and shoes on. By the time she stands up, she is ready to go for her walk. Since the weather is nice today, she will be walking outside. On cold or rainy days, she prefers to exercise to a video in her family room. Total time spent from her bed to her front door is three minutes. She chose not to brush her teeth or hair yet today, which usually adds an extra two minutes.

Maggie's friend Christine is waiting for her in front of her house. They both do a few minutes of stretching before starting their walk. Maggie and Christine have three different walking routes that they like to use. Each one is approximately 3 miles, which is a distance both ladies have found to be satisfactory for them. Today it is Christine's turn to choose which route to use and she picks the one with the most hills.

After approximately 40 minutes, Maggie is home. She goes into the kitchen, pours herself a large glass of water and eats a banana. She then moves into the family room to stretch and do a few toning exercises with her hand weights. This takes approximately 15 minutes. The next thing she does is put a star on her calendar to indicate that she exercised today. Maggie keeps her activity calendar in the bathroom so she sees it several times each day as a gentle reminder.

At the end of each month, Maggie tallies up all of her stars. She writes the total on the bottom of the page before flipping to the next month. When she has a month with very few stars, she thinks back to figure out why. She works to overcome these obstacles the next month and sets her goal to earn more stars. She tends to notice that the more stars she has accumulated, the less stress she seems to have in her life.

It is now 7:00 A.M. Maggie showers. Just before getting out of the shower, she turns the water temperature to cold for an invigorating, 30-second cold water blast. She does this to help stimulate her blood flow and to help invigorate her mind. She doesn't mind that the cold water also helps keep her hair nice and shiny as well. Maggie gets dressed and ready for the day. Her family is now up and her house is bustling with movement. She eats breakfast with her family. Then she packs her lunch, plus three snacks to take with her to work. She fills up her water bottle, which holds 4 cups of water, with water and ice. After taking the kids to school, she is on her way to work. She drinks all of the water, through a straw, before arriving at work at 8:30 A.M.

Maggie's Workday

At 10:00 A.M., Maggie notices that she is getting a little hungry. She takes a short break and eats half of the sandwich that she packed for lunch. She knows that the protein from the tuna will help keep her alert while she continues to work on her project.

She breaks for lunch at 12:30 P.M. She eats the majority of the lunch that she packed, eating slowly and really enjoying it. She then decides to take a short walk around the block for some fresh air and to help clear her head for the afternoon. This walk takes 10 minutes. Maggie is back at her desk with five minutes to spare. She closes her eyes and takes several deep breaths. She is now ready to work again.

At 3:30 P.M. she takes a bathroom break and takes the banana with her from her lunch bag. She eats the banana on her way to the bathroom, returning to her desk to work until 5:00 P.M.

Maggie's workday is over. She collects her belongings and stops to fill her water bottle at the drinking fountain. She proceeds to her car, which she parked four blocks away from work on purpose. She is tired and does not feel like walking to her car, but she has no choice.

On her drive home, she gets stuck in heavy traffic. She is starting to get hungry and is anxious to get home. When the traffic comes to a standstill, she reaches into her lunch bag and pulls out a snack bar. She eats it and drinks her water to prevent herself from becoming overly hungry and making a poor choice, such as stopping at a fast food drive-through.

Maggie Returns Home

When she gets home her dog, who is excited and needs to go outside, greets her. She quickly walks Fido around the block, then proceeds to make dinner. She planned her dinner menu the night before based on the food that she had available, to avoid making impulse decisions about what to prepare.

She makes sure to include extra vegetables in the dinner meal because she didn't eat many during her workday. While she prepares the meal, she sips on a glass of water, again using a straw. This is her tenth and final cup of water for the day. She finds that if she drinks much after dinner her sleep is interrupted by the need to use the bathroom.

She eats slowly with control during supper. She stops eating when she is no longer hungry, even though there is still a small amount of food left on her plate. After cleaning the kitchen and watching her favorite television program, Maggie decides that she would like something sweet to eat. She thinks back about the day and realizes that she ate four servings of fruit, meaning that she has had plenty. She opts to eat a frozen fudge bar, which is chocolate and satisfying, yet very low in fat and calories.

Three hours later, Maggie gets ready for bed. She then takes her multivitamin with a small amount of water. Although she knows that her diet is balanced and healthy, she takes the vitamin as a safety net for any vitamins that she may not be getting quite enough of. She sets her alarm clock, allowing for eight hours of sleep, and places it on the bathroom counter. She again lays out her exercise clothes because tomorrow she is planning to use her "mama time" to do an exercise video in her family room.

She does 20 leg lifts with each leg to the side, followed by 20 back kicks with each leg while she brushes her teeth. This is a habit that she formed years ago when she was not making time for regular exercise in her life. Now she just routinely does the leg lifts as she brushes her teeth every night.

Summary of Maggie's Activity

Maggie walks with her friend every Monday, Wednesday, and Friday morning. On Tuesday and Thursday mornings she either does an exercise video or rides her bike. Saturday is the day that she likes to dance and jump around with her kids for 30 minutes to music. Sunday is her official day off from exercise, although she sometimes goes for a walk or a bike ride with her family.

At work, she takes a 10-minute walk around the block during her lunch break on the days when the weather is pleasant. On rainy days, she often walks up and down a few flights of stairs to increase her heart rate during her lunch hour. She also avoids the elevator at work and in public buildings and always looks for the stairs.

Maggie routinely parks her car at least four blocks away from work. When she goes shopping, she also parks at the far end of the parking lot. Maggie looks for any opportunity to move her body that she can find. She considers herself to be an active person.

Summary of Maggie's Diet

Maggie, like most thin people, finds that feeding her body well makes her feel and look great. She eats a combination of 8 to 10 servings of fruit and vegetables each day. She always drinks at least 8 cups of water per day. She limits her intake of sugar, saturated (animal-based) fat, and refined, processed foods.

She eats something within the first hour of waking and then continues to feed her body small, frequent meals and snacks, every three to four hours all day long. She almost always stops eating prior to feeling uncomfortable. She does not like to eat after 8:00

P.M., as she does not like to go to bed with much food left in her stomach.

Maggie finds that when she is eating healthy foods, her body craves even more of these foods. When she used to eat processed, high-fat foods, these were the foods that her body seemed to crave. She finds that as she gets older, she is more concerned with feeding her body well to prevent cancer, heart disease, adult-onset diabetes, osteoporosis, and obesity. She is attempting to defy the aging process.

Summary of Maggie's Sleep Pattern

Maggie knows that her body needs approximately seven hours of sleep to function at its peak. When she gets six hours or less, she does not have the energy to exercise and finds herself using caffeine to help her through her day. She is also less likely to make healthy food choices on these days. Her body seems to crave more fat and fried foods.

She also notices that on the days when she goes to bed early or sleeps late and gets more than eight hours of sleep, she is more sluggish, again making poor activity and eating choices. She has learned this through trial and error. Her wellness triangle seems to be perfectly balanced with a total of seven hours of sleep every night.

Balance, Variety, and Moderation

The diet that you choose to follow for the rest of your life needs to be balanced, varied, and likeable. You calmly choose foods that are nutritious most of the time and don't feel great guilt over consuming foods that you don't consider "healthy." All foods can fit into your daily diet. Do not be tempted to ever go back on a restrictive "diet." Losing weight slowly is the key to permanent weight loss.

Your attitude will determine your success. You need to learn to love and accept yourself, and praise yourself for your progress. Remember, as you get closer to your goal weight, the fat will come off more slowly. Chasing that last 5 pounds for the rest of your life may not be worth it. Don't be too hard on yourself if you do overeat occasionally. Overeating one day and undereating the next is all a part of the normal eating experience. Trust yourself to balance it out by following your appetite and listening to your body.

Chapter 14:
Summary of Steps to Follow to Become a Thin Person

1. Observe the way thin people eat
2. Mimic a thin person's eating style.
3. Think and live as if you already are the thin person you are destined to become!

CHAPTER 15

Recipe Alterations and Menu Ideas to Get Started

Low-fat cooking does not have to mean bland, tasteless food.

Plan Ahead

To avoid eating on impulse or frying up the same old quick burger and fries, plan one week at a time and write down your menus. This will help prevent you from panicking at mealtime and ordering pizza.

You don't need to get overly specific, just choose an entree and a vegetable for each meal you prepare. For most people, it will be the evening meal, which happens to be the time of day when people tend to deviate from their healthy eating goals. You can always add a vegetable salad or fruit side to any meal.

Next, make sure you have all of the ingredients available. If you are planning to make lasagna tonight to eat tomorrow evening, read through your recipe to make sure that you can stop by the store ahead of time to pick up missing ingredients. Don't forget to make sure your fruit bowl is stocked and that salad fixings are always handy.

Check your schedule to see if you have any activities that may prevent you from having enough time to cook a certain meal. If you have other commitments, consider making a meal that cooks itself in the crockpot. Weekends are a great time to do any grocery shopping and prep work for your upcoming week of meals.

The key to healthy meals with variety is planning ahead. Don't wait until suppertime to decide what you should make. If you are a busy family with different schedules, planning meals in advance will also help simplify your life. Even if you are unable to all sit down together as a family every night, at least you know that a good meal is always prepared and ready to eat.

What to Make?

The beauty of following the *THIN CHOICES* program and mimicking the eating habits of thin people is that you can truly eat anything you like. You do not need to give up all of your favorite high-fat foods. All you need to do is simply revise your recipes and pay attention to your hunger and satiety signals to determine how much to eat.

This chapter includes low-fat recipe alterations that you can use in almost any of your recipes. Of course, you will have a handful of recipes that should not be altered because the low-fat substitutes cause the quality of the finished product to suffer significantly. For those recipes, such as homemade chocolate chip cookies, you may find that limiting the quantity you consume is your best option.

All of these low-fat substitutions have been tested repeatedly. The finished product you are making will not suffer in appearance or in taste. Eating, after all, is one of the greatest pleasures in this world. Why waste that precious little space in your stomach with food that is just mediocre, even if it is low-fat or healthy?

> "If a food or recipe doesn't taste good, I won't eat it."
> —Ann H.

There are four easy steps to low-fat cooking.

1. Purchase low-fat ingredients.
2. Use low-fat preparation techniques.
3. Make low-fat substitutions in your recipes.
4. Record your recipe changes.

1. Purchase low-fat ingredients.

Most fruit and vegetables are naturally fat free. Fruit and vegetables are an important part of a healthy diet that promotes weight loss and helps prevent disease. Those that do contain fat, such as avocados and olives, contain heart-healthy fats and should not be avoided.

Buy low-fat and nonfat dairy products such as skim milk, nonfat sour cream, light cream cheese, and low-fat yogurt. Cheese suffers in taste when the fat has been removed, so you may prefer to just limit your intake of cheese instead of using a reduced-fat variety. Or choose a naturally lower fat cheese, such as mozzarella (half the fat of cheddar) for your recipes.

When purchasing meat, choose items that have the words "loin" or "round" in them, as they are the leanest choices. Poultry, fish, and seafood usually contain less fat than red meat. Just remember to remove the skin from the poultry prior to eating it.

Most grains, such as wheat, rice, and oats are also naturally low in fat. The prepared grain items are those that have added fat, such as muffins, granola, croissants, and rice pilaf, just to name a few. Pasta, although lacking as a significant source of nutrition, does not contain much fat provided you follow the serving sizes.

The fat and oil category is very calorie dense and usually loaded with fat. The items included in this category are oils, butter, stick and tub margarine, mayonnaise, salad dressings, lard, bacon, and bacon grease. Your initial goal is to choose the fat sources that are the least taxing on your heart. These include cooking spray, vegetable oils, and other fats that are as close to a liquid at room temperature as possible, such as tub margarines. The fats that are very artery clogging and taxing on the heart are lard, bacon, bacon grease, butter, stick margarine, and other animal sources of fat. The fats that are solid at room temperature cause the most damage to our arteries. Oils that are hydrogenated have been pumped full of hydrogen, producing trans-fatty acids, which are just as taxing to the heart as cholesterol, and therefore should also be limited or avoided.

Omitting the fat sources in your recipes is the simplest solution for decreasing the fat content in all of your recipes. The only problem is that your entire recipe will be changed if you do not replace this omitted fat with a substitute. We will discuss the best fat substitutes next.

2. Make low-fat substitutions.

You can make many low-fat substitutions as long as you have the low-fat substitute when you need it. For example, if you need to make a birthday cake but don't have yogurt available (an excellent substitute), you may find yourself reverting back to using oil. Keeping the common replacements available will help you more easily transition your recipes.

A list of low-fat food substitutes that you will probably use daily follows. Once you get the basic low-fat cooking techniques down, you will find that you can alter just about any recipe. You will no longer be stuck making the same recipes out of the one low-fat cookbook that you own. You will even be able to take Aunt Elsie's famous stroganoff recipe and bring it to your new, healthy table. Don't be afraid to experiment.

You can also save calories by decreasing the sugar in your recipe by ¼ to ½ of the requested amount to decrease the calories in your finished product.

Low-fat ingredients to substitute in healthy cooking to reduce fat, saturated fat and cholesterol

Instead of:	Substitute this:
1 whole egg	2 egg whites or ¼ cup egg substitute
1 cup butter (rice or pasta dishes)	1 cup chicken broth
1 cup oil (baked goods)	1 cup yogurt or pumpkin or 1+½ cups applesauce
Oil (to stir fry)	cooking spray, wine, or chicken broth
1 cup oil (in a marinade)	1 cup wine, fruit juice, or nonfat Italian dressing
1 cup whole milk	1 cup skim milk
1 cup light or heavy cream	1 cup evaporated skim milk (shake well)
1 cup sour cream (vegetable dips)	1 cup nonfat sour cream 1 cup plain nonfat yogurt or 1 cup nonfat cottage cheese + 2 tsp lemon juice, blended
1 cup cheddar cheese	1 cup mozzarella or ½ cup cheddar cheese
Cream cheese	light cream cheese, nonfat cream cheese (cheesecakes only)
Mayonnaise	reduced fat or nonfat mayonnaise
Salad dressings (for salads)	use the dipping technique or reduced fat salad dressing

Ground beef

Brown, drain, and rinse your ground beef (with hot water) before adding it to your recipe. This decreases the fat contained in the beef by 50 percent without sacrificing its flavor. This works well for all dishes that are based upon browned ground beef: chili, lasagna, tacos, burritos, stroganoff, stuffed peppers, or pasta sauces. Just remember to add your seasonings after you've rinsed the beef.

Start with the leanest ground beef available when making a recipe where the beef is not browned first, such as hamburgers, meatballs or meatloaf. Greater than 90 percent lean is best. Blotting your meat with a paper towel helps soak up some of the fat if you don't use lean meat. Be aware that ground turkey is sometimes higher in fat than lean ground beef because dark meat and skin may be added.

Fat content comparison of ground beef

Serving size is 3½ ounces (size of a deck of cards)

Ground beef—70 percent lean	calories	fat grams
Broiled patties	243	18.0
Broiled patties, after blotting	230	15.7
Pan-broiled crumbles, drained	195	11.7
Pan-broiled crumbles, drained and rinsed	135	6.1

Ground beef—80 percent lean	calories	fat grams
Broiled patties	228	15.2
Broiled patties, after blotting	217	13.8
Pan-broiled crumbles, drained	191	10.9
Pan-broiled crumbles, drained and rinsed	130	5.3

Ground beef—95 to 98 percent lean	calories	fat grams
Lean ground round, all	115	3.5

Making Pasta Entrees with Cheese

When you make pasta dishes with cheese (such as lasagna), substitute a nonfat cottage cheese for most of the cheese that is normally included in the middle of the dish. Use half of the amount of cheese that you would normally use on the top. Substituting mozzarella for all or part of the cheese in the recipe also decreases the fat by half.

Your lasagna will still taste wonderful, but the fat content will be much lower. By placing the majority of the hard cheese on the top, your dish will *look* like a full-fat entree. After all, we do eat with our eyes!

Thin People Eat Soup

Studies have shown that individuals who start their meal with soup eat fewer overall calories at the meal that follows. Soup eaters consumed from 200 to 350 fewer calories than those who didn't eat soup. If you ate soup as an appetizer just two times each week, it would create a calorie deficit that would produce a 6- to 11-pound weight loss in one year. No wonder soup diets are so popular!

Many people who have gone too long without eating will become overly hungry, feeling slightly anxious about getting some food into their stomach. Soup takes the edge off of this overstimulated appetite quickly. Remember, the alternative tends to be a trip through the fast-food drive-through. Start thinking soup!

"I enjoy eating soup. It fills me up without adding a lot of calories."
—Beth L.

All of the thin people who were interviewed stated that they consume soup on a regular basis. The majority avoid cream- and cheese-based soups because of the excessive fat content. Most thin people prefer tomato- or broth-based soups.

Many thin people also report eating soup as a main course a couple of times each month. They usually included bread and a fruit with their soup. Just think of the calorie savings at these meals!

Soup can be as easy as opening a can and warming up the contents. The big advantage of canned soups is convenience as well as having the nutrition label so easy to access. You can instantly tell how many calories and how much fat is in each serving. The disadvantage of canned soup is that the sodium content is often high. This means that you'll need to drink extra water and avoid weighing yourself the next day because of the water-weight gain.

Making homemade soup can also be quite simple and quick. A broth base is the lowest in fat content. Add as many vegetables as you like without any concern about adding extra fat. Put your cooked vegetables into a blender and puree to thicken the soup without the fat. Use lean meat or skinless chicken breast to add protein without too much extra fat. Any excess fat will float to the top and can be skimmed off once it is chilled.

When ordering soup from a restaurant, remember that the tomato- and broth-based soups are the healthiest, whereas the creamed and cheese soups are much higher in fat content. Be aware of any meat is that is added (sausage contributes the greatest amount of fat).

3. Use low-fat preparation techniques.

Low-fat cooking techniques include baking, broiling, steaming, grilling, or roasting. The main cooking techniques to avoid are frying and broasting, which is deep-frying under pressure. You can bake your favorite fried foods in the oven, which will decrease the fat content by at least half.

To bake your fried favorites, simply toss the item in a plastic bag that contains a beaten egg white. Next, roll your pieces into finely ground, seasoned breadcrumbs or croutons. Then arrange your pieces in a single layer onto a cooking sheet that has been lightly coated with vegetable oil cooking spray. Lightly spray your pieces with the cooking spray to help them brown nicely. Bake your food at 350 degrees for anywhere from 7 to 40 minutes, depending on what you are oven-frying. Potatoes that have been cut into French fries will take the longest, whereas cheese curds will be done the quickest. Remember to watch your cheese curds closely, as the cheese begins to ooze quickly.

Telling you how to make your favorite fried foods lower in fat does not mean that you can now eat unlimited portions of oven-fried cheese curds without any consequences. It means that you aren't forbidden from eating any of your favorite foods while you continue to lose weight. All foods can be modified to be lower in fat content, but moderation with all foods is still a must.

4. Record your recipe changes.

Have a stack of 3-by-5 index cards available in your kitchen. When you begin to revise a recipe, take one of the cards and write down the ingredients you are using. Measure each of the ingredients and indicate the fat content of the items that you use. This will help you determine the number of fat grams in each portion. Don't forget to write down how you are cooking it, including the oven temperature and length of cooking time.

Once your family has tasted the recipe, make comments on the bottom of the card. Your comments might say that the lasagna has 9 grams of fat in one-twelfth of the recipe; it stuck to the bottom of the pan and needed more salt. Now you will know that the next time you make this recipe, you will want to spray the bottom of your baking dish with cooking spray, put some of the tomato sauce into the pan before the noodles, and add more salt or other spices to the meat sauce while cooking.

If you do not record your recipe alterations and comments, all you will remember the next time you plan to make lasagna is that your family complained about the quality. You may fall back on the tried and true way you know everyone loves. Then, instead of sharing a meal with your family, you will be eating a card-board-tasting frozen diet meal with a portion size meant for a three-year-old.

Revising recipes takes a little bit of work initially, but since the average family rotates the same 8 to 10 meals through their dinner menus, it won't take you long to perfect your favorites. You will find all of your effort to be well worth it when your jeans are getting loose and your energy level starts to skyrocket.

Concerns Some People May Have

You may worry that you are depriving your family of good tasting food. Your food will still be very tasty. If you find that you have revised a recipe to the point where it doesn't taste good any-more, then your comment on the bottom of your recipe card will say so. The next time you make that recipe, you will know to add some fat back into the dish. Try not to have the all-or-nothing mentality when improving your cooking and recipes.

You may also be concerned that you might be depriving your children or already thin mate of the fat their bodies need. Chil-dren under the age of two do need extra fat to help their brains grow, which is why most doctors recommend breast milk or baby formula for the first year of life and then whole milk until they are two. You can always add extra fat or calories to your child's food on his or her own plate if you feel extra fat for growth is needed.

Most people compensate for a lack of fat in their diet with larger servings of food. This is especially true for growing teenag-ers and extremely thin adults who burn excessive calories throughout the day. Again, you have the option of putting sour cream, butter, or shredded cheese on the table for each individual to add as they desire if you are concerned.

The childhood and teen obesity rate is greatly increasing ev-ery year. Currently, two out of three Americans are either obese or overweight. We would all be wise to begin decreasing the added fat in the diet of our families at home to help slow this trend.

When you serve one of your low-fat recipes to others, you will anxiously await their feedback. But resist the urge to blurt out that it is a "low-fat, healthy" recipe. Whenever people are told they are eating something that is "good for them" or low fat, they instantly think it tastes bland or not as good as the original.

Once I served an excellent, low-fat mocha chocolate cheesecake at a family gathering, and someone said, "I suppose Jill's dessert is fat free again!" To which I responded, "No, just a regular cheesecake." When the whole cheesecake was devoured, several people asked for the recipe. They were amazed to find out that it was made with nonfat cream cheese and nonfat cottage cheese. Each slice had only 100 calories and 4 grams of fat, as opposed to the usual 450 calories and 28 grams of fat per slice!

Have fun cooking and don't take it too seriously. Some of the best recipes take several revisions to perfect. Bon appétit!

Chapter 15:
Summary of Steps to Follow to Become a Thin Person

1. Make low-fat substitutions to all of your favorite recipes.
2. Record the low-fat changes you have made right on your recipe card.
3. Choose soup for a meal or appetizer a few times each week.

CHAPTER 16

Summary of the *THIN CHOICES*™ Program

There are two vicious cycles.

Which Life Cycle Do You Currently Fit Into?

Most people will fall into one of two daily life cycles. The first one, which is where a lot of overweight individuals will fit, is called the poor choices/feel bad daily life cycle. This is the life cycle where the majority of choices that are being made every day cause the person to feel bad.

The nutrition choices typically being made by a person in this life cycle include making poor food choices, usually consuming excess fat and calories. This person will probably eat with little regard to hunger and satiety sensations. Intake of fruit, vegetables, and water is usually low.

Activity levels of the person in the unhealthy choices life cycle are low. This person does not engage in regular exercise sessions and limits calorie-wasting activities. This person often spends more time viewing television or computer screens than the person not in this cycle. This person will feel tired and sluggish due to inactivity. Sleep is neither sound nor consistent for most individuals in this cycle.

The person in this poor choice life cycle is usually carrying excess body fat. His or her energy level will be low and their stress level may be high. This person may feel depressed and sometimes even out of control. He or she does not enjoy family, friends, and work accomplishments as he or she once did.

See the diagram below to figure out if you are currently in this unhealthy/feel bad daily life cycle.

The second life cycle is called the *THIN CHOICES*/feel good daily life cycle. This is the cycle where the daily choices that are being made for nutrition, exercise, sleep, and stress-reduction cause the person to feel good.

The person in this cycle is typically eating in relation to hunger and satiety signals. He or she is consuming fruit, vegetables, and water in sufficient quantities, and limits the intake of excess

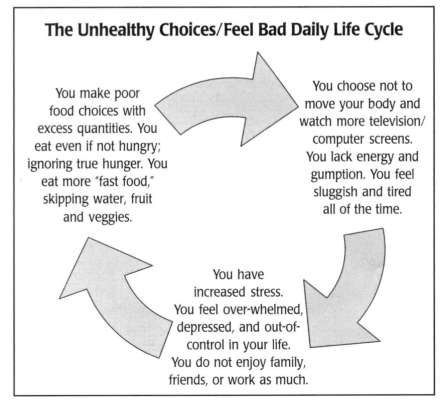

The Unhealthy Choices/Feel Bad Daily Life Cycle

You make poor food choices with excess quantities. You eat even if not hungry; ignoring true hunger. You eat more "fast food," skipping water, fruit and veggies.

You choose not to move your body and watch more television/computer screens. You lack energy and gumption. You feel sluggish and tired all of the time.

You have increased stress. You feel over-whelmed, depressed, and out-of-control in your life. You do not enjoy family, friends, or work as much.

fat and calories.

In this cycle, the person often engages in regular exercise sessions, classifying him- or herself as an active person. He or she often has enviable energy levels without relying on stimulants for pep. This person usually sleeps soundly through the night.

Life feels in control for this person with minimal stress. This person will also appear more optimistic than the person in the unhealthy life cycle. This life cycle is usually full of people who do not carry large amounts of excess body fat. Compare your habits and energy level to the diagram below to see if you fall into this cycle.

> "One of my best weight-loss tips is to give up the TV—in other words, get off your butt!"
>
> —Mary Jo B.

The THIN CHOICES/Feel Good Daily Life Cycle

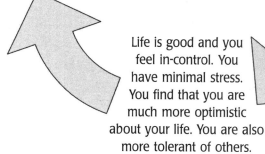

You make good food choices. You eat when hungry and stop when satisfied. You limit "fast food" and "trigger foods." You consume plenty of water, fruit and veggies.

You are moving your body most days of the week for at least 30 minutes. You are experiencing an increase in energy. You feel strong and full of life.

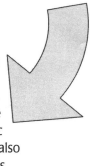

Life is good and you feel in-control. You have minimal stress. You find that you are much more optimistic about your life. You are also more tolerant of others.

Are You Stuck in the Wrong Cycle?

Most people will find that they definitely fit into just one of the above two life cycles, both of which are vicious. It seems that the more positive choices that you make, the more positive choices your body craves. The more unhealthy choices you make, the more unhealthy choices your body craves.

To move away from the unhealthy daily life cycle, you need to make the to-

> "I keep my weight under control by exercising three to four times per week and eating what I want in moderation."
>
> —Lisa G.

tal commitment to all areas of your life. Remember that your body will start to desire more of the choices you predominantly make. It will become easier with repetition. As soon as you start to experience the increased energy and improved attitude, the healthier choices will be much more desirable.

THIN CHOICES Simply Summarized

The *THIN CHOICES* program teaches you how to raise your metabolism by adding some foods, omitting others, changing the size and timing of meals, as well as gently altering lifestyle habits. Most importantly, you are learning how to listen to your body and feed it accordingly.

A few of the healthy items you have added to your diet include water, fruit, and vegetables. They are all essential to maintaining optimal fluid status and to provide low-fat, high-fiber foods, which have been proven to promote weight loss. You are also eating more lean protein. Food items you have limited or omitted are high-fat foods and empty calories. More of your food choices are found in nature than in a factory.

The portion size of each of your meals and snacks should now be limited to the size of your fist, which is approximately the same size as your stomach. Waiting no longer than four hours between eating sessions is the ideal way to keep your metabolism working and burning calories all day long.

Activity requirements for an optimal metabolic lift include: moving your body for a total of 30 minutes most days of the week, plus weight training two to three days per week. The more you choose to move your body, the faster you will see results.

Listening to your body and its appetite and satiety signal is the final skill you have begun to learn in following the *THIN CHOICES* program that will help you achieve your weight-loss goals. Since your lifestyle and mind-set have changed as you have adopted this program, your weight loss will be a permanent change as well.

> "The older I become the more I watch my diet and weight for my health instead of just trying to maintain that perfect size six!"
>
> —Mary Jo B.

If you are only able to make one or two of these positive lifestyle changes in the beginning, that is all right. As you build upon this foundation and begin adding new healthier habits, you will begin to see your body transform more quickly. Once again, you do not need to be perfect in all of your daily choices, just aim to be "pretty good most of the time."

All Chapters:
Summary of Steps to Follow to Become a Thin Person

1. Resist the urge to ever go on another restrictive diet.
2. Eat something for breakfast within the first hour of waking up every day.
3. Eat something as soon as you notice you are hungry.
4. Stop eating as soon as you notice you are no longer hungry.
5. Leave some food on your plate at one meal every day.
6. Carry healthy snacks with you at all times.
7. Stop eating at least two to three hours before going to bed.
8. Eat 8 to 10 servings of fruits and vegetables every day.
9. Practice the dipping technique, with all sauces on the side.
10. Limit your intake of fat to 30 to 40 grams per day for a woman and 40 to 50 grams per day for a man.
11. Eat a snack or light meal before going to a restaurant or party.
12. Avoid or limit your personal trigger foods.
13. Drink a minimum of 8 cups of water every day.
14. Move your body for at least 30 minutes most days of the week.
15. Lift weights two to three days per week.
16. Breathe deeply for five minutes twice each day.
17. Breathe deeply while exercising or playing.
18. Make low-fat substitutions to all of your favorite recipes.
19. Choose soup for a meal or appetizer a few times each week.

CHAPTER 17

Maintenance of Weight Loss

Reaching your weight-loss goal is just the beginning.

Congratulations! You have finished reading this book and you are well on your way to reaching your weight-loss goals. You are probably wondering what you should do once you do reach your goal. Maybe you are now fitting into what you consider your "skinny jeans" or maybe you are just at a point where you finally feel good in your skin again. Whatever your end goal is, when you do reach this goal, it is really only the beginning.

It is the beginning of your life as a thinner you. You will not be going back to the old eating habits and sedentary lifestyle that got you into trouble in the first place. You are going to continue making the same lifestyle choices that you have been making during the course of your weight loss. These choices should now be habits and feel more like a way-of-life for you than a restrictive diet.

> "I think these high-protein diets are out of control. To lose weight permanently, you don't need a diet, just a healthier lifestyle."
>
> —Anne Y.

Begin to Dress to Flatter Your Thinner Body

As you have been losing weight, you have probably been noticing that your clothes are looser. Maybe you have even been showing off your baggy pants to friends with comments like: "Hey! There's room for both of us in here now!" Yes, this is fun, but if you don't begin to purchase more fitted clothes, you may eventually start to fill them out again.

This has happened with several of my weight-loss participants. They don't purchase new clothes as they want to wait until they reach their ultimate weight-loss goal, but then pretty soon they are allowing themselves a few too many treats. They are still content, because they still have excess room in their clothes, but eventually they may return to their previous poor lifestyle choices.

This is not to say that you need to buy an entire new wardrobe each time that you lose 10 pounds. You may just buy a new pair of blue jeans. Jeans are fitted and an excellent indicator of your body shape changes. You may also decide to give away your oversized sweatshirts and stretch pants. Eventually you will start tucking your shirts into your pants.

> "Instead of weighing myself, I like to monitor my body size by how my jeans fit."
>
> —Heidi N.

For an impartial judge of what you should be wearing, according to your body size and assets, ask a department store attendant for help. You may not be able to make these decisions for yourself, as your mind may still be telling you to cover up. At first you may feel uncomfortable, but as you start to receive compliments, you will know that you are dressing more flattering.

Thin Clothing Techniques

Dressing monochromatically, or wearing only one color, will give you the illusion of height. Most people find dark colors, such as black or navy blue, to be the most slimming. Long skirts will help slim thick legs and also give the illusion of height. Wearing high-heeled shoes provides length to short legs.

A lot of women who are not quite at their goal body size have commented that having their hair done nicely with makeup applied helps boost their confidence. By wearing nice jewelry or placing a colorful scarf around your neck, you will also be drawing the eye of on-lookers up.

Learning how to dress to flatter your body shape will help accentuate your positive assets and camouflage any less than desirable areas. Don't be afraid to ask a clothing consultant for assistance. Sometimes it is just a matter of finding the right style or fit for you.

Attitude over Body Size

Your attitude will ultimately reflect how you feel about yourself. Your weight is just your body's pull against gravity or a number on the scale. Your blue jean size is just a number on a little tag in the back of your pants that most people will never see. What others do see when they look at you is your attitude about yourself.

The ultimate icing that gives thin people their enviable position in our society is good posture combined with confidence. When a person walks into a room standing fully erect with their head held high, they possess confidence. We all want to know what their secret is. They automatically appear to "have it all together." They look successful, happy, and thin, even if they are carrying some excess body fat.

> "I find that by standing up straight and feeling like I am thin and beautiful, I appear to be more attractive. How you feel and portray yourself is half of your image."
>
> —Jill R.

Weight-loss professionals will report the illusion of a 5- to 10-pound weight loss when a person has good posture. Practice holding your head high with your shoulders back and walk tall. Pretend that you are royalty when you walk into a room and then observe those around you who are watching your entrance.

Smile and look as if you are happy, even if you do not feel happy at that moment. If you are shy, fake having the confidence you envy. Soon you will begin believing you are a happy, confident person. You may notice that others are willing to overlook your body imperfections when you appear confident and comfortable in your own skin.

Learn How to Accept a Compliment

You have undoubtedly received at least a few compliments about your appearance in the past few months. How did you react to these observations? Were you gracious and appreciative or did you shoot the compliment—and its giver—down?

Many people who have been overweight for several years will be shocked when the compliments start coming. They will be taken aback and may deny the compliment is true. They may say, "Yes, but I sure have a long way to go!" This will make the person who gave the compliment feel uncomfortable. Even if you think you are just being modest, it will be perceived as negative.

When you receive your next compliment, realize that someone is noticing you look good. By merely saying, "Thank you," you will be validating that person's opinion, yet not sounding vain or conceited. You may want to practice repeating "thank you" several times before the first time you may actually need to use it.

What to Do If You Start to Regain Weight

First, stop and take a deep breath. Take a look at what has changed in your lifestyle choices. Have you started to fall back into your old, unhealthy patterns of eating and inactivity? Ask yourself which daily life cycle you are currently in. Now ask yourself which daily life cycle you want to be in.

Second, take charge of your life again. You only need to remain accountable to yourself. Get out your lifestyle diary or notebook and record everything you put into your mouth. Analyze your intake as if you were a registered dietitian. By now, you know which items may be missing from your diet or which ones are being consumed too frequently.

The third step is to begin recording your exercise sessions on your calendar again. This is the best method of tracking your exercise and is quite motivational. If you have been exercising and recording your activities on the calendar, you may need to increase the frequency or the duration of you sessions.

> "I try to focus on how I feel when I'm eating well and exercising. I am much happier when I feel strong, healthy, and slim."
> —Heidi G.

Fourth, examine your self-talk. Which inner voice are you listening to? You have a little chubby guy in a red suit on your left shoulder and a thin and fit angelic figure dressed in white on your right shoulder. They are both whispering in your ears. Which one you choose to listen to is up to you. Think about it. Which one is really your friend?

Last, make sure that you are not feeling guilty about the daily choices that you do make. Focus on what you did do well each day, not on the areas where you may have relaxed your focus for the day. Emphasizing the positive choices will help keep your overall attitude positive.

> "If you 'cheat,' get over it! Don't dwell on it."
> —Jenny M.

Visualize your path to becoming thin as if it were a road that you are traveling along on a trip to your favorite destination. How long it takes you to reach your destination will determine how many traffic jams and detours you encounter, as well as how many shortcuts you may find. Think of the less healthy choices as the detours that will make your journey a little longer whereas the healthy choices you make are the shortcuts. Every choice you make will determine how long it will take for you to reach your goal. You do need to continue making pretty good choices most of the time in order to maintain your new thinner self, but by the time you reach your goal, most of your healthy choices will be habits.

The mind is a powerful tool. It has been said that "where the mind goes, the body will follow." Believe that you are a thin person; begin living like a thin person and soon you will become that thin person.

SUMMARY OF
COMMON CHARACTERISTICS OF
ALL THIN PEOPLE SURVEYED:

- They thought they should eat more fruits and vegetables than they actually did most days.
- They stopped eating several hours before going to bed.
- Most did not eat again after their evening meal.
- They went to bed with their appetite rated between neutral and hungry.
- They preferred to eat fish, chicken, and seafood instead of red meat the majority of the time.
- They all considered themselves to be active people.
- They avoided or limited fried and processed/refined foods.
- They incorporated their favorite, high-fat foods into their diet in moderation, avoiding the feeling of deprivation.
- They monitored their body size more by how their clothes fit than by the scale.
- They decreased their total food intake and exercised more if they noticed they had gained some weight.
- They avoided buying and keeping their out-of-control foods at home.
- They attempted to eat slowly and really taste their food.

SUGGESTED READING LIST

Anderson J. W., E. C. Konz, R. C. Frederich, and C. L. Wood. Long-term weight-loss maintenance: a meta-analysis of US studies. *The American Journal of Clinical Nutrition*, 74 (5), 579–584, 2001.

Bell A. B. and B. J. Rolls. Energy density of foods affects energy intake across multiple levels of fat content in lean and obese women. *The American Journal of Clinical Nutrition*, 73 (6), 1010–1018, 2001.

Breathnach, S. B. *Simple Abundance: A daybook of comfort and joy.* New York: Warner Books, 1995.

Brownell, K. D. and T. A. Wadden. Etiology and treatment of obesity: Understanding a serious, prevalent and refractory disorder. *Journal of Consulting and Clinical Psychology*, 60 (4), 505–517, 1992.

Collage Video: Exercise and fitness videos. Call 800-433-6769 for a free catalog or visit www.collagevideo.com.

Danforth, E. and E.A.H. Sims. Obesity and efforts to lose weight. *New England Journal of Medicine,* 327 (27), 1947–1948, 1992.

Dove dark chocolate. The inside wrapper contains a positive affirmation; the chocolates have only 4 grams of fat per piece!

Drapeau, V., J. Despres, C. Bouchard, L. Allard, G. Fournier, C. Leblanc, and A. Tremblay. Modifications in food-group consumption are related to long-term body-weight changes. *The American Journal of Clinical Nutrition*, 80 (1), 29–37, 2004.

Fairburn, C. *Overcoming Binge Eating: Proven effective in clinical research.* New York: The Guilford Press, 1995.

Fletcher, A. M. *Thin for Life: 10 keys to success from people who have lost weight and kept it off.* Shelburne: Chapters Publishing Ltd., 1994.

Foreyt, J. P. and W.S.C. Poston. The role of the behavioral counselor in obesity treatment. *Journal of the American Dietetic Association*, 98 (10), S27–S30, 1998.

Gavalas, E. *Yoga Minibook for Weight Loss: A specialized program for a thinner, leaner you.* New York: Simon and Schuster, 2003.

Greene, B. and O. Winfrey. *Make the Connection: Ten steps to a better body— and a better life.* New York: Hyperion, 1996.

Kaul, L. and J. Nidiry. High fiber diet in the treatment of obesity and hypercholesterolemia. *Journal of the National Medical Association*, 85 (3): 231–232. 1993.

Kornfield, J., S. Salzberg, and S. Young. Beginner's Mind: 3 classic meditation practices especially for beginners (audiocassettes). Sounds True Publishing, 1999.

Kratina, K., N. L. King, and D. Hayes. *Moving Away From Diets: New ways to heal eating problems and exercise resistance.* Lake Dallas: Helm Seminars Publishing, 1996.

Lahti-Koski, M., P. Pietinen, M. Heliovaara, and E. Vartiainen. Associations of body mass index and obesity with physical activity, food choices, alcohol intake, and smoking in the 1982–1997 FINRISK Studies. *American Journal of Clinical Nutrition*, 75 (5), 809–817, 2002.

Ornish, D. *Eat More, Weigh Less: Dr. Ornish's life choice program for losing weight safely while eating abundantly.* New York: Harper Collins, 1993.

Pawlak, L. *Appetite: the brain body connection.* Hermosa Beach: JEBLAR INC., 1995.

Pawlak, L. *Stop Gaining Weight: Three "no nonsense" steps to no more pounds.* Hermosa Beach: JEBLAR INC., 2001.

Ponichtera, B. J. *Quick and Healthy Cookbook, Volume I: For people who say they don't have time to cook healthy meals.* The Dalles: ScaleDown Publishing, 1994.

Ponichtera, B. J. *Quick and Healthy Cookbook, Volume II: More help for people who say they don't have time to cook healthy meals.* The Dalles: ScaleDown Publishing, 1995.

Redmond L. *Feel Good Naked: 10 no-diet secrets to a fabulous body.* Gloucester: Fair Winds Press, 2002.

Rinke, W. J. *Make It a Winning Life: Success strategies for life, love and business.* Rockville: Achievement Publishers, 1992.

Rippe, J. M. and S. Hess. The role of physical activity in the prevention and management of obesity. *Journal of the American Dietetic Association*, 98 (10), S31–S38, 1998.

Seligman, M. Learned Optimism: How to change your mind and your life (CD audio book). New York: Simon and Schuster, 2001.

Sell, C. *A Cup of Comfort for Inspiration: Uplifting stories that will brighten your day (and temporarily take your mind off of food)*. Avon: Adams Media Corporation, 2003.

Siler, B. *The Pilates Body: The ultimate at-home guide to strengthening, lengthening, and toning your body—without machines*. New York: Broadway Books, 2000.

Stallings, S. F. and P. G. Wolman. Effective weight maintenance techniques of healthy, normal-weight, middle-aged women. Topics in Clinical Nutrition, 7 (3), 56–62, 1992.

St. James, E. *Simplify Your Life: 100 ways to slow down and enjoy the things that really matter*. New York: Hyperion, 1994.

St. James, E. *Simplify Your Life with Kids: 100 ways to make family life easier and more fun*. Kansas City: Andrews McMeel Publishing, 1997.

Tolle, E. *The Power of Now: A guide to spiritual enlightenment*. Novato: New World Library, 1999.

Warren, R. *The Power to Change Your Life: Exchanging personal mediocrity for spiritual significance*. Grand Rapids: The Encouraging Word, 1998.

THE *THIN CHOICES* EPIPHANY

One day you decide you're not happy
with the body you call home,
As you look around, feeling cheated;
you complain, envy, and groan.
Then you figure out that it's all about choices,
You start to change how you talk to yourself,
hearing new inner voices.
Now you are good to your body and rewarded with pride,
As your thinner self emerges facing challenges in stride.
Embracing life you regret waiting so long,
Your heart is so light and happy it sings a sweet song.
Thank you, thank you, to the heavens above,
You are finally at home in a body
you now unconditionally love.
Congratulations!

—Jill M. Fleming, MS, RD

INDEX

A

Alcohol
    diuretic effect of 74
    impact on weight loss 64-65
    impact on sleep 90
Allergies, food 1
American Cancer Society 43
Attitude, and importance of for
    success 11-12, 123-124
    over body size 123-124

B

Basal metabolic rate (BMR). *See*
    metabolism
Bedtime, eating before 41-42
Binges, and trigger foods for 68
Bloating 46
Blood sugar 19, 56, 65, 69
Body composition, monitoring
    changes in 12-13
Body size, attitude over 123-124
Breads 56
Breakfast, importance of eating 15-
    18
    best time for 17

C

Caffeine 16, 90
    diuretic effect of 74
Candy 56. *See also* M&Ms
Carbohydrates 56
    complex 56
    sensitivity to 69
    simple 56
Cereals 56
Characteristics, common of thin
    people 127
Cheese, pasta with 109
Chicken Lasagna, recipe, fat grams
    52
Children, teaching healthy eating to
    37-38
Clean Plate Club 29-38
    Break the Chain illustration 35
    eating and physical signals 34
    eating too quickly 30-31
    mindless eating 31
Clothing, dressing in flattering
    122-123
Coffee 16
Compliment, acceptance of 124
Cooking low-fat 103-113
Cravings, psychological 22

Give the Gift of
Thin People
Don't Clean Their Plates
to Your Friends and Colleagues

CHECK YOUR LEADING BOOKSTORE OR ORDER HERE

❑ **YES**, I want _____ copies of *Thin People Don't Clean Their Plates* at $22.95 each, plus $4.95 shipping per book (Wisconsin residents please add $1.53 sales tax per book). Canadian orders must be accompanied by a postal money order in U.S. funds. Allow 15 days for delivery.

❑ **YES**, I am interested in having Jill Fleming inspire my employees or organization. Please send information.

To learn more about the THIN CHOICES concepts or to purchase lifestyle diaries and fat revealer guides, log on to <u>www.ThinChoices.com</u>.

My check or money order for $_____ is enclosed.

Please charge my: ❑ Visa   ❑ MasterCard
                    ❑ Discover   ❑ American Express

Name _____

Organization _____

Address _____

City/State/Zip _____

Phone_____ E-mail _____

Card # _____

Exp. Date_____ Signature _____

Please make your check payable and return to:
Inspiration Presentations Press
P.O. Box 3372 • LaCrosse, WI 54602-3372

Call your credit card order to: 866-482-1159
Fax: (608) 782-2074 • www.ThinChoices.com • Email: Jill@thinchoices.com